Good Hearted Guidance
THE HEALTHY WAY

THE HEALTHY WAY

Weight Loss Wisdom and Lifestyle Solutions

Cheri Bianchini, RN, BSN, PHN

Dedicated to the unlimited source
of love and radiant health
that lives within all of us.
Let it grow and shine.

To the memory of my late husband, Jerry,
who remains an everlasting reminder
of unconditional love
and my continued wellspring of faith.

In honor of Cheladee,
my daughter, my teacher,
my friend.

Photo Credits

Walnut photo courtesy of Walnut Marketing Board,
c/o Torme & Company, San Francisco, CA.

All other front cover photos by Rick Ruggles.
Found Heart™ Photographs © 2002
Visit his website at **www.rickruggles.com.**

Back cover photo by Jana Marcus, Santa Cruz, CA.
Book cover and interior design by Marianne Wyllie, Santa Cruz, CA.

All inquires should be addressed to:
The Healthy Way Inc.
3251 Mission Drive
Santa Cruz, California 95065

Visit our website at **www.thehealthyway.us**

Disclaimer
The ideas and suggestions contained in this book are not intended as a
substitute for medical advice. Before embarking on any diet or exercise
program, including those presented in this book, it is advisable to consult
with your physician.

ACKNOWLEDGMENTS

If one word could summarize my feelings about the completion of this work, it would be gratitude. I wish to thank the following individuals for their talent, intelligence and loving support…

Donna Williams-Smith who offered the initial spark to ignite this project and who kept the flame going with her faithful encouragement. Gracias Amiga!

Marianne Wyllie, graphic designer extraordinaire, thank you for all the love and laughter you brought along the way in bringing this book into existence. We had so much fun, I want to write another book so we can continue working together!

Bonnie Jo Bell, my mentor for twenty five years (and former Iowa State Spelling Bee Champion), you could have a career in proofreading! Thanks for your keen eyes and beautiful heart. I love you dearly.

Blessings to Maia Farrell, my sweet neighbor and angel in disguise, who offered the impetus for the book cover concept and who led me to the incredible photography of Rick Ruggles…thank you, thank you, thank you! And special thanks to Deena Saroyan for the walnuts!

A heartfelt thanks to Rick Ruggles, "Heartographer" beyond compare and a true kindred spirit. You have captured so many hearts and spread such love with your amazing talent. I will forever remain in awe.

Lisa Foster, my dear friend, thank you for always being so giving of your time, energy and exceptional ability to make everything you touch look beautiful. Your artistic counsel on this project has been greatly appreciated.

Thanks to Maya Barsacq, Maren Jacobsen, and Cynthia Harvey for the many hours you assisted me in pouring over these pages.

To the wonderful staff at **The Healthy Way**, my deepest gratitude for "holding down the fort" and allowing me the time and space for projects such as this book.

I wish to offer my appreciation and respect to all the past and present clients of **The Healthy Way** program, who have shared their souls so freely and provided enormous inspiration for the content of this collection. Many blessings to you!

To my beloved friends, I give you all a big hug for loving me, listening to me, and most of all, believing in me, even when I haven't. Your friendship adds to my creativity and makes life worth living.

I am honored and grateful to the people of Santa Cruz County, who read my column and who write back with words of praise and encouragement.

Last, but certainly not least, to that universal power greater than ourselves… thank you for giving me the opportunity to serve.

Heart-Shaped World

The shape of a heart is a universal symbol that stands for LOVE.
As simple in design as a circle or square, the heart is different from
other forms in that it evokes an emotion. For centuries, its shape has
been a spiritual insignia of trust, caring and goodwill toward
others. I have a special affinity with the heart shape; my eyes
have become attuned to its form. I often come upon heart-
shaped objects in nature, be it rocks, a tomato slice in
my salad, or the white patch of fur on my black
dog's chest. Whenever they appear before me, I
feel a deep connection and a state of grace
with life. I chose to use the image of
heart-shaped food throughout this
book, as a reminder of the love
that surrounds each and
every one of us,
sometimes in the
most unexpected
of places!

INTRODUCTION

SINCE 1986, late at night after the little one has been tucked into bed, I have sat at my kitchen counter, taken pen in hand and have written a weekly column that appears in several local Santa Cruz, California publications. Focusing on health, nutrition and positive lifestyles, the columns started as a temporary advertising strategy for my business, **The Healthy Way.** I received such overwhelmingly positive feedback from the public that now, years later, I continue with the same format and appreciate having been told my newspaper column decorates the front of many refrigerators!

This is a collection of work that spans almost 20 years as a weight loss counselor and 40 years as one who has intimately lived with weight and body image issues. These pages encompass professional observations, personal insights and a large volume of accumulated reference materials. Not just another "how to" book, *The Healthy Way* is a practical, user-friendly guide to living more consciously. The goal is to have you live its content, use it and pass it on.

In years past, I have wrestled with the question…What is the highest value, what belief is the most important to live by? As a nurse I've witnessed the ravages of disease. In the last five years, personally, I have seen most of my own family die, beginning with my sweet husband. Unequivocally, I have learned from experience that, without health, all other values cannot be realized. Love, peace, truth, wisdom…none of these virtues can be fully appreciated without first having health.

Certainly, we have no control over some aspects of life and I believe we must be at peace with this fact, since it appears to be an integral part of life's mystery. However, in many areas of our lives, we have enormous power, such as the food we choose to eat, what we think and how we care for our bodies.

I find it a great honor to be a positive force in people's lives and if you incorporate even one of the tips outlined on these pages, my goal will have been achieved. There truly are so many simple ways we can all help to nourish our hunger for love, connection and optimal health. May this book serve to supply some of the answers.

Thank You and Treasure Yourself.

Cheri

Cheri Bianchini

TABLE OF CONTENTS

FOOD FACTS

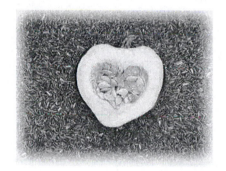

Blood Sugar Stabilization
The Path to Health

FOR ALMOST TWO DECADES, **The Healthy Way** has promoted blood sugar stabilization as a major key in weight loss and optimal health. Basically what the term refers to is maintaining a balance between glucose (blood sugar) and insulin levels within the body. By doing so, weight and body fat content typically stay within normal limits; energy levels remain constant; cholesterol and triglycerides fall within the norm; cardiovascular health is strong and the body can function optimally. When the blood sugar levels are continually out of balance, accelerated aging and numerous degenerative health hazards can occur.

The following is a guide, listed in order of importance, to maintain a stable blood sugar level:

Balanced Eating
What this means is you don't fly out the door with a piece of white bread toast as a meal that is expected to carry you until the afternoon. Ideally, a meal should consist of the major macronutrients:

- Protein (meat, fish, poultry, dairy, soy)
- Carbohydrates (fruit, vegetables, whole grains, beans, rice)
- Fats (butter, olive oil, flaxseed oil, avocado, seeds and nuts)

An "on the run" balanced breakfast could include 1 or 2 slices of whole grain toast (such as Ezekiel bread) with 1tsp. almond butter spread on top, 1 or 2 hard boiled eggs, or a carton of nonfat plain yogurt with a handful of strawberries.

Instead of a hot dog and fries for lunch, have a Chef's salad with chicken or fish on top (tofu if vegetarian); ask for the dressing on the side and use half the amount.

The cornerstone of **The Healthy Way** food plan is choosing foods of a "low glycemic index." This refers to foods that have a low to mild effect on insulin response. For instance, a donut can trigger the pancreas to release an excess of insulin, whereas a bowl of old fashioned oatmeal may cause a much slower, lesser amount of insulin to be excreted.

A balanced diet is actually a cleaner, more simple way of eating and is not difficult to implement once you get the basics down and have detoxified from the standard American diet. Contrary to popular belief, simple sugars such as white flour, white sugar and processed foods are not essential to the diet and do not belong to any of the food groups.

Frequency of Eating

The most common problem I've been confronted with, as a nutritional counselor is meal skipping or following irregular eating habits. By doing so—

A. Blood glucose levels drop due to lack of food

B. The body must get more glucose for brain functioning

C. Gluconeogenesis occurs by breaking down muscle to create new glucose for the brain

D. Adrenaline and cortisol—the stress hormones are stimulated and as a result, the pancreas will secrete more insulin at the next ingestion of food to counteract the presence of these chemicals.

Researchers at Georgia State University found that active people who ate infrequently stored unburned calories as fat and decreased their metabolism. If the irregular skipped meal patterns continue, year after year, this constant overproduction of insulin may contribute to a state of hyperinsulinemia, insulin resistance, Type II diabetes and cardiac disease. By eating four to six regular small meals throughout the day (such as breakfast, lunch, dinner, mid morning and mid afternoon or evening snack) insulin levels will be lowered and blood sugar stabilization will occur.

Weight Loss and Decreased Body Fat

Obesity has been shown to play a role in insulin resistance, especially if the body fat is concentrated around the abdomen (apple shape). With excess body fat, cells can be less sensitive to insulin's message (insulin resistance) and energy from food is stored in the fat cells rather than burned.

Without question, I know the weight-challenged individual often eats less than their thinner counterpart and is more likely to gain weight than a lean person. Why?? Because fat people and thin people respond to the release of insulin differently. By eating a low glycemic food plan at regular intervals, the result is insulin and blood sugar become balanced. Dietary and lifestyle changes can be difficult to implement all at once, so keep in mind the "tortoise won the race." Staying focused on steady progress will result in a lifetime of improved health and weight control.

Exercise!!

It doesn't matter what type of movement it is, be it aerobic, resistance, flexibility exercises, or working vigorously in the garden, a regular program of exercise has been shown to reduce insulin levels and reverse insulin sensitivity. As stated before, insulin resistance refers to a reduced sensitivity to insulin and in response the body must secrete an increased amount of the hormone. Research has confirmed when higher levels of insulin are repeatedly required, diabetes, heart disease, hypertension, and now even cancer are being linked to hyperinsulinemia. Over 60 million Americans have insulin resistance. Regular exercise, even of moderate intensity, helps lower blood sugar levels, balances out insulin and offers numerous health enhancing benefits.

Limit Intake of Stimulants

If coffee were the only stimulant used today, that would be one thing…but it isn't. Nicotine, caffeine, diet pills, and many of the popular "thermogenic" products on the market which contain Ephedra (Ma huang), all raise insulin levels. With regular use, the biological toll of accelerated aging and degenerative disease are greatly increased. Although alcohol is known to be a depressant, many people experience a state of stimulation from the ingestion of the chemical ETOH. Alcohol is broken down as pure glucose and causes the blood sugar level to dramatically elevate and drop, resulting in fluctuation. The goal is to keep these levels balanced.

Reduce Stress

All of the hormones in the body are affected by the stress response (including insulin). Long ago the "fight or flight" syndrome helped our ancestors deal with survival, which is no different than today. The problem, though, is today we deal with more constant adrenaline rushes, from traffic jams to the food we eat. Continued stress weakens the body by causing a state of dis-ease. For normal functioning, the body's hormones should be in balance.

Blood Sugar Evaluation

	OCCASIONALLY TO FREQUENTLY	RARELY TO NOT AT ALL

Do you experience:

*1. Thinking of food (sense of hunger) obsessively	❏	❏
*2. Lightheadedness	❏	❏
*3. Cravings for sweets or carbohydrates	❏	❏
*4. Drop in energy (body feels like "lead bricks"), especially mid day	❏	❏
*5. Tunnel or blurred vision	❏	❏
*6. Headache	❏	❏
*7. Difficulty in concentration	❏	❏
*8. Indigestion or gas	❏	❏
*9. Rapid weight gain or difficulty controlling weight	❏	❏
*10. Out-of-control or compulsive behavior with food, especially sweets and starches	❏	❏
*11. Mood swings/depression	❏	❏
*12. High cholesterol or triglyceride readings	❏	❏
13. Hunger between meals or snacking late at night	❏	❏
14. Cold extremities	❏	❏
15. Consumption of processed or packaged foods	❏	❏
16. No breakfast and/or irregular meals	❏	❏
17. Drinking 2 or more cups of coffee, tea, sodas or artificially sweetened beverages per day	❏	❏
18. Alcohol consumption more than once per week	❏	❏
19. Snacks generally consist of fruit, crackers, chips, cookies or candy	❏	❏
20. PMS/menopausal symptoms	❏	❏
21. Take birth control pills or female hormone replacement therapy	❏	❏
22. Bread, pasta, or other starch, fruit or sweets are usually included in one or more meals per day	❏	❏
23. Smoke one or more packs of cigarettes per day	❏	❏
24. Experience stress at both home and work	❏	❏

TOTALS

A score of 4 or more classic symptoms indicated by (*) or an overall score of 10 or more "occasionally to frequently" items suggests that you may suffer from blood sugar fluctuation.

WATER

INCREDIBLE AS IT MAY SEEM, water is one of the most important factors for losing weight and keeping it off. Many of us take water for granted, but it may be the only true "Magic Potion" for permanent weight loss.

Water suppresses the appetite naturally and helps the body metabolize stored fat. Studies have shown that an increase in water intake can actually reduce fat deposits. Here's why: The kidneys can't function properly without enough water. When they don't work to capacity, some of their load is dumped onto the liver. One of the liver's primary functions is to metabolize stored fat into usable energy for the body. But if the liver has to do some of the kidney's work it can't operate at full throttle. As a result, it metabolizes less fat, more fat remains stored in the body, and weight loss stops.

The overweight person needs more water than the thin one. Larger people have larger metabolic loads. Since we know that water is the key to fat metabolism, it follows that the overweight person needs more water. Water helps to maintain proper muscle tone by giving muscles their natural ability to contract and by preventing dehydration. It also helps to prevent the sagging skin that usually follows weight loss—shrinking cells are buoyed by water, which plumps the skin and leaves it clear, healthy and resilient. Water helps rid the body of fat. During weight loss, the body has a lot more waste to get rid of; all that metabolized fat must be shed. Adequate water helps flush out the waste.

How much water is enough? On the average, a person should drink eight 8-ounce glasses every day. That's about 2 quarts. However, the overweight person needs one additional glass for every 25 pounds of excess weight. The amount you drink also should be increased if you exercise briskly or if the weather is hot and dry.

DRINK GREEN TEA

BEFORE YOU ORDER ANOTHER CAFE LATTE or gulp down more diet soda— instead, think about switching to a cup or two of green tea. After 20 years of research, the health benefits are now clearly defined. All tea contains polyphenols (antioxidants such as vitamin A, C, E and the mineral, selenium) which act to cut down the activity of cell damaging molecules known as free radicals. Free radical formation has been blamed in the development of heart disease, cancer and other serious ailments.

Green tea, in particular, contains epigallocatechin gallate (EGCE), which is the most potent antioxidant yet discovered! One cup a day is beneficial; however, for maximum protection, studies suggest that it's best to drink 4 cups per day.

Because green tea undergoes less processing than black tea, it contains twice the polyphenols and about ⅓ less caffeine. Research published by the *International Journal of Cancer* and the *American Journal of Clinical Nutrition* demonstrated that green tea aids with the following:

- *lowers blood pressure and inhibits blood clotting*
  Studies have shown that an individual's risk of heart disease and stroke can be cut in half!

- *interferes with cancer cells*
  By rendering cellular DNA resistant to mutation, growing evidence suggests that green tea prevents cancer cells from forming and inhibits the growth of tumors already in existence.

- *enhances immunity*
  Green tea boosts the activity of key immune system fighter cells. Patients undergoing chemotherapy can especially benefit.

- *facilitates digestion*
  It does so by encouraging the growth of beneficial bacteria in the intestine and by controlling levels of glucose in the bloodstream.

- *prevents tooth decay*
  Levels of dental plaque can be reduced by holding green tea in the mouth for a few seconds.

People who drink green tea on a daily basis have unusually low rates of heart disease and cancer. They also live longer. And unlike other antioxidants, those in green tea cause no toxic side effects. It should be noted that Dutch scientists recently found that the anticancer effects of green tea were reduced more than 90% when dairy products were added to it. The bottom line—it's green tea time everyone!

The Truth
About Soft Drinks

PERHAPS MANY OF YOU ALREADY KNOW that by pouring a cola-type drink on your windshield in a snow storm, you will prevent the glass from freezing. If you are troubled by unsightly toilet bowl stains, pour in a can of Coca Cola and one hour later; flush those stains right down the drain. It's amazing!! Got a rusted nut, bolt or a corroded battery terminal? Not a problem… a little dab of cola, either regular or diet, will fizz them clean within minutes.

Most people wouldn't think of drinking such products as "Mr. Clean" or "Windex," yet when it comes to cola (a proven effective household solvent), the average American gulps down more than 800 cans per year! Yes, it may taste good, but it's killing us!!

The bubbles and fizz in soft drinks are caused by phosphoric acid and carbon dioxide. The phosphorus in the acid upsets the body's calcium-phosphorus ratio and dissolves calcium out of the bones, eventually resulting in osteoporosis. Carbon dioxide is a waste product exhaled by the lungs, but if ingested back into the system, it depletes our bodies of oxygen, when cola drinks are consumed.

Soft drinks are acidic compounds. In order to neutralize a 12 oz. can of cola, it takes 32 glasses of high pH alkaline water. It is well known in the medical profession that disease, particularly cancer, flourishes in an acidic, low oxygen environment. Soft drinks create both.

Cola drinks also contain caramel coloring, which together with phosphoric acid have been shown to cause birth defects. A study done in Japan where 100 pregnant mice were fed a diet high in both agents, yielded 40 deformed fetuses.

Soda pop is the #1 item in the American diet that contains the most sugar. Regular soft drinks use predominantly cane syrup or high fructose corn syrup as the sweetener. The average 12 oz. Coke has 150 (empty) calories and about 10 teaspoons of sugar per serving...that's more than 1 oz. of sugar per can!! Any wonder why diabetes is skyrocketing?

Nutra Sweet and Equal, the artificial sweeteners used in the diet versions of soft drinks, may pose even greater health risks. Clearly, children have absolutely no business eating or drinking anything artificially sweetened...the documentation is a mile long and more than conclusive!

Every kid knows a dirty penny returns to its original copper luster when soaked in cola. Place an extracted baby tooth in the same solution and within a few days, it will totally dissolve...which makes it tough on the tooth fairy!! Rats who were otherwise well fed, but given nothing to drink except cola beverages, had their molar teeth dissolved down to the gum line within 6 months time.

Sadly enough, soft drinks are the number one beverage of choice, followed by coffee. Whatever happened to water?? One trick that works is to make a goal of drinking 8 glasses of water or herbal tea before any sodas can be consumed.

The Los Angeles School District has banned the sale of soft drinks at schools as of 2004. This will create a $3-million budget deficit, as Coke, Pepsi and others pay for placement of these very profitable vending machines. Let us salute the L.A. school board for their forward thinking and courage in allowing health rather than the almighty buck to preside. May other school districts follow their stance.

THE FIVE WORST FOODS

A FTER YEARS IN THE NUTRITION BUSINESS and even more years studying human health, I've come to believe that the following foods should be consumed with caution. Here's my top five hit list.

1. **Aspartame:** Artificial Sweetener marketed as "NutraSweet" or "Equal." It's found in diet drinks, diet desserts, sugarless gum, even some children's vitamins! When the temperature of Aspartame exceeds 86° F., the wood alcohol in aspartame converts to formaldehyde and then formic acid, which in turn causes metabolic acidosis. There are more complaints called into the FDA regarding artificial sweetener than any other additive. More than 5000 products contain aspartame. Pregnant women and children absolutely should not ingest aspartame.

2. **Genetically Engineered Foods:** 60 to 75% of all non-organic supermarket foods now test positive for the presence of genetically engineered ingredients. Mounting scientific evidence suggests that G.E. foods (or genetically modified organisms—"GMO") present serious hazards for human health and the environment. The FDA and the federal government are presently not required to label G.E. foods. We should be allowed to know what we are eating!

3. **Nitrites & Nitrates:** Found in most smoked, processed meats, especially bacon, sausage and hot dogs. These substances become highly carcinogenic in the body.

4. **Hydrogenated & Partially Hydrogenated Fats:** Also known as "Trans-fats," the body doesn't recognize them or process them correctly and thus, this toxic substance is stored in the tissue. Throw the margarine out and switch to organic butter, but use it in moderation.

5. **The White Stuff:** Sugar and white flour are both highly processed and devoid of all vitamins, minerals, enzymes and life force. Allergies, obesity, diabetes, cancer can all be attributed to the "white stuff." We need to cut way back on its consumption.

One way to omit or limit these five items from the diet is to buy organic and read the labels. You will be healthier as a result!

BUTTER VS. MARGARINE

HYDROGENATION IS A MAN-MADE TECHNIQUE of adding a hydrogen ion to a liquid oil, thus creating a solid product such as margarine or Crisco. The problem with this fifty-year-old technology is that it changes the molecular structure from a "cis fatty acid" to a "trans fatty acid," causing a potent carcinogenic reaction. Hydrogenation clogs arteries and elevates cholesterol levels as well.

Worse yet, it has been shown to not break down in the body. Listed as hydrogenated or partially hydrogenated in many of our baked goods, processed foods, cereals, crackers and frozen meals...the food industry uses this product because it's cheap, it increases flavor and flakiness and extends shelf life. It can be easily reused, as in the case of fast food french fries which may be cooked in two week old hydrogenated shortening. The bottom line is to try and limit your exposure to hydrogenated and partially hydrogenated products as much as possible. Many health advocates believe that organic butter, in small amounts, is better for one's health than shortening and margarine.

The overall goal is to cut down on all fats. In baking, substitute unsweetened applesauce in lieu of the fat. Switch to an all fruit jam for your toast. Tahini or hummus spreads are also good. Use a non stick pan when frying. Saute with water, broth, wine, spray-type vegetable oils or soy sauce. When reading labels, look at the type of fat being used, not just the percentage. All fats are not created equal! Beware of the words "hydrogenated" and "partially hydrogenated" and look for products without these poisons in them.

All fats and oils should be stored in the refrigerator to avoid rancidity. Extra virgin expeller pressed (or cold pressed) olive oil or flaxseed oil is good for cold use, i.e., salad dressings and marinades. Peanut oil, grapeseed oil and butter are best to cook with because they have a higher heat tolerance and won't break down as readily as other fats.

It's all the little steps we take that make a big difference. The bottom line is...butter is better than margarine, because it's natural.

GMOS

A N ENORMOUS DEBATE OF GREAT SIGNIFICANCE IS IN FULL SWING regarding the dietary use of GMOs (genetically modified organisms) or GEOs (genetically engineered organisms). Yet according to a 1999 study by Consumer Reports, fewer than a third of U.S. shoppers know anything about it. What is genetically engineered food? It's a laboratory technique that changes the DNA of living organisms and alters its biochemical process to enhance certain commercial characteristics. For example, to make tomatoes more frost resistant, scientists have inserted a gene from the fish, flounder, that is believed to help the tomato survive in cold weather.

Promoters tell us GMOs are the greatest scientific advance of our time...that world hunger could cease to exist! Critics warn that genetic engineering is a risky, unpredictable technology, capable of creating a public health crisis and irreversible biological pollution of vast proportion. Many countries across the globe are fighting to be biotech-free zones. The European and Japanese food industries are refusing GMO exports from the U.S., unless these products have been segregated and clearly labeled.

Over 60% of processed foods in America contain genetically engineered ingredients and the FDA currently does not require disclosure of such in labeling. The primary GMO foods include: soybeans, corn, potatoes, tomatoes, peanuts, canola and cottonseed oils, and milk with bovine growth hormone. Products such as Kelloggs Corn Flakes, Similac Baby Formula, Duncan Hines cake mixes, even Garden Burgers have all tested positive for GMO ingredients.

Here's my question...if scientists are still in the midst of a raging debate whether GMO foods are safe or not, why then do they fill our grocery shelves in such abundance? Furthermore, why isn't the U.S. required to label GMO foods when parts of the world flat out refuse to eat them? Don't we have a right to know what we put into our bodies?

Choosing certified organic foods is the best way to ensure avoidance of GMO foods. Cut down on processed foods and low-budget products because they are more likely to be affected. Read labels and especially avoid non-organic soy based ingredients such as soy flour, soy oil, lecithin and hydrolyzed vegetable protein.

For more information call 1-800-Real Food, visit **www.safe-food.org** or **www.truefoodnow.com.**

LIFE IN THE FAST FOOD LANE

FOR MOST PEOPLE, THE GREATEST NUTRITIONAL PROBLEM with typical fast foods is the number of calories. A quarter-pounder with cheese, fries and a shake contains about 1,130 calories!

You may find the following fast food recommendations on how to lower your fat and caloric intake helpful:

- Order a hamburger (not a cheeseburger) without the mayo and you may strip away 135 calories and 15 grams of fat.

- Wipe the tartar sauce off your fish sandwich and save a third of the calories and almost two-thirds of the fat.

- Always choose the low calorie or "lite" salad dressings.

- Don't use those handy packets of croutons and chow mein noodles and save about 50 calories each.

- When ordering hotcakes, go easy on the butter and syrup. Better yet, skip the butter.

- Order ham for the breakfast sandwich and hold the sausage and bacon.

- A bagel with cream cheese has as much fat as a bagel with ham, egg and cheese. Order the plain bagel instead of the cream cheese and save 100 calories and 10 grams of fat.

- Choose a biscuit, muffin, or bagel over a croissant or Danish.

- Choose barbecue, honey, or sweet and sour sauces instead of Ranch dressing or tartar sauce and save 18 grams of fat, more than you'd get in an order of onion rings (and go easy on all the sauces).

- Order a chicken fajita instead of cheese enchiladas.

- Order a taco salad, hold the guacamole and sour cream, and don't eat the fried shell. Amazing example: Taco Bell Taco Salad with Salsa: 850 cal./52gm. fat. Taco Bell Bean Burrito: 370cal./12gm. fat.

- A bean burrito has as many calories as a serving of nachos, but only half the fat and saturated fat.

- If you just can't bring yourself to skip all the cheese, ask for cheese on only half of the pizza.

- Choose half a chicken breast over a thigh and a drumstick.

- If you've just got to eat some skin, order Original Recipe Fried Chicken instead of Extra Crispy.

Food Facts ❤

KNOW WHAT YOU'RE EATING!

THE MANUFACTURERS OF PROCESSED FOOD are in business to make money, not necessarily to offer healthy, wholesome cuisine. With the fast paced lives we all lead, sometimes there is no choice but to indulge in these convenience foods. Be sure to check the label's ingredients and percentages to be an informed consumer.

Contadina Alfredo Sauce. A typical four-ounce serving contains 34 grams of fat, 20 of them artery-clogging saturated fat. That's like drowning your pasta in more than a third of a stick of butter. If you want a good bottled pasta sauce, try Millina's Finest Spaghetti Sauce. It's sugar-free and no fat is added.

Taco Bell's Taco Salad with Shell. With the shell, the platter of beef, cheese and beans has 14 teaspoons of fat, more than 5 teaspoons of saturated fat, and 905 calories. That's almost all the fat and saturated fat an adult should eat in an entire day. If you're in the mood for a fast food salad, head to McDonald's. Their Chunky Chicken Salad contains a single teaspoon of fat and ¼ teaspoon of saturated fat.

Oscar Mayer Lunchables.™ It would be hard to invent a worse food than these combos of heavily processed meat, artery-clogging cheese, and mostly white-flour crackers. The line averages 5 ½ teaspoons of fat (that's 55% of calories) and 1,517mg of sodium. You'd get less fat and salt from two thin slices of Pizza Hut's Pepperoni Pan Pizza.

Stouffer's Entrées. Despite their popularity, Stouffer's entrees get a greater percentage of their calories from fat (44%) than any other major line of frozen dinners or entrées. Not one of Stouffer's 52 varieties meets our criteria for a "healthy" frozen meal. If you want low-sodium, low-fat frozen meals, try Tyson Healthy Portions, Healthy Choice Dinners, or Le Menu New American Healthy. Fran's Healthy Helpings has a line of frozen dinners just for kids.

A WORD ABOUT SUGAR

Linus Pauling, the late Nobel prize winning scientist, as well as many others, believe that sugar is the true culprit in our diet and a major factor in the fattening of America. In just 200 years, our consumption has risen from an average of 3 lbs. per year to a startling current average of 125 lbs. per year. Worst yet, the average American teenager consumes over 175 lbs. per year, generally in the form of sodas. Only 25% of the sugar in our diet is added at the table. The other 75% of that is sweetener hidden in our food.

125 pounds of sugar a year is equivalent to:

- Over 17,969 jelly beans per person per year.
- Over 1229 12-oz. cans of regular cola per person per year.
- Over ¼ lb. of sugar a day.
- An extra 32 teaspoons of sugar a day.
- An extra 630 calories every day!

Other Names for Sugar:

Maltodextrin	High fructose syrup
Corn sweetener	Sucrose
Fructose	Dextrin
Invert sugar	Sorbitol
Maltose	Corn syrup
Raw sugar	Molasses
Maple sugar	Cane sugar
Brown sugar	Honey
Malt syrup	Glucose
Dextrose	Confectioner's sugar
Lactose	Turbinado sugar

LABELS
WHAT DO THEY REALLY SAY?

UNFORTUNATELY FOOD LABELING IS NOT AN EXACT SCIENCE and, in fact, can often be misleading rather than helpful in your search for healthy foods. The common listing of "sugar" is only one example of how confusing this subject can be. When assessing the amount of sugar in a product, make sure you spot all the sugars listed; they come in many forms. Sucrose indicates only white refined table sugar. As previously mentioned, glucose, fructose, brown sugar, corn syrup and honey are also forms of sugar. These are listed separately from sucrose on labels. Added together, sugars may be more abundant than you think.

If a product is labeled "sugar free" or "sugarless" it cannot, by FDA standards, contain either sucrose or any other form of sugar. Only low-calorie sweeteners such as saccharin and aspartame are allowed. Chewing gum is the exception. It can be called "sugarless," even though it may contain sorbitol, a sugar alcohol that has as many calories as sucrose, but does not promote tooth decay. However, the FDA requires that these "sugar free" labels also include such disclaimers as, "not for weight control" or "useful only in preventing tooth decay."

- A low fat food has 3 grams or less of fat. Foods with low saturated fat contain 1 gram or less.
- A low sodium food has 140mg or less. A very low sodium item contains 35mg or less per serving.
- Low cholesterol means 20mg or less of cholesterol and also 2gm or less of saturated fat.
- Low calorie foods have 40 calories or less per serving.
- Lean meat or poultry must contain less than 10gm of fat, 4.5gm or less of saturated fat and less than 95mg of cholesterol per serving.

When you see the words "reduced fat" on the label—Beware! Check the calorie count, sugar and carbohydrate content. Typically, manufacturers compensate for the lower fat by adding more sugar and carbohydrates to maintain flavor.

"LICKS, NIBBLES AND TASTES"
THE SNEAKY CALORIES

D O YOU LICK THE CAKE BATTER OFF THE BEATER? Sample a fingerful of dough? A smidgen of coconut? Licks and nibbles do add up:

Cake batter:

1 licked beater	=	13 cals.
1 licked bowl	=	38 cals.

Cookie dough:

1 fingerful	=	80 cals.
1 licked bowl	=	80 cals.

Frosting:

1 licked beater	=	30 cals.
1 licked bowl	=	30 cals.

Pie Crust:

1 nibble	=	14 cals.

Garnishes:

1 licked jam knife	=	4 cals.
1 pinch coconut	=	9 cals.

Bagel:

½ dry bagel, no topping	=	200 cals.

Orange juice:

1 12oz. glass (unsweetened)	=	6 small oranges

Chicken nugget:

1 1oz. nugget	=	80 cals.

Scone (700 cals.) equivalent to all of the following:

an english muffin spread with jam, a dish of cherries, a bowl of corn flakes with banana, two slices of light toast with marmalade, cup of fruit cocktail and a bowl of oatmeal with sliced peaches.

How to Avoid Pesticides

I T IS NOW CLEAR THAT FOODS WITH PESTICIDE RESIDUE can have a toxic effect. Washing off our produce with water rarely cleans it sufficiently. Those who live in an area abundant with organic fruits and vegetables have a choice. However, for some people, especially families on a budget, organic produce becomes cost prohibitive. Still others may not even be aware of the level of residual pesticides in their food.

The chart below will help guide you to make wiser organic *vs.* nonorganic produce choices. For example, I always buy organic strawberries, rather than commercial strawberries, because of their high residual pesticide rate. Commercial avocados on the other hand are less dangerous because of their low rating.

Residual Pesticide Rating

Scale: 0=Lowest   100=Highest

Strawberries (1 cup)	100	Potato (1)	60
Cherries (U.S. 1 cup)	88	Celery (1 stalk raw)	50
Apples (1)	88	Tomatoes (½ raw)	50
Cantaloupe (Mex. 1 cup)	80	Green Beans (½ cup)	50
Apricots (4)	80	Cucumbers (½ cup raw)	45
Pears (1)	78	Grapes (1 cup)	45
Raspberries (1 cup)	78	Bananas (1)	30
Spinach (½ cup)	77	Carrots (1 raw)	20
Peaches (1)	72	Green Peas (½ cup)	20
Melon (U.S. 2 cups)	72	Broccoli (½ cup)	18
Grapefruit (½)	71	Cabbage (½ cup raw)	18
Bell Pepper (½ raw)	70	Brussels Sprouts (½ cup)	18
Squash (½ cup)	70	Sweet Potatoes (1)	8
Cherries (import; 1 cup)	68	Corn (½ cup)	5
Blueberries (1cup)	68	Green Onions (¼ cup raw)	5
		Avocados (½)	2

Source: "A Shopper's Guide to Pesticide in Produce" Environmental Working Group, a Washington D.C. based consumer group. For more information: **www.ewg.org**

Battle on the Home Front

Since September 11, 2001, we have been bombarded by every form of the media with reports of recent terrorist attacks and threats of biological warfare by anti-American forces. It seems to me, a destructive plot aimed at harming U.S. citizens has been in effect for years now…chemical contamination in the form of artificial, supersized, sugar ladened, processed foods. They line the shelves of our grocery stores and fast food outlets. Vending machines in schools across the nation dispense this junk daily to our youth. Well disguised as clowns and cartoon characters, they act as spokespeople selling our kids on their products at an early age.

These food "impostors" are known to decrease health and make us gain weight. Since 1970, the percentage of Americans considered obese has increased 60%, resulting in a medical crisis of untold proportions. Obesity costs the U.S. $99.2 billion dollars per year, creating significant financial concern as well. How can we fight back????

Step one is to decrease our exposure to these harmful agents in the diet by limiting their consumption, thus sending a much needed message to the manufacturers that "we aren't going to take it anymore!" Secondly, we as a nation need to get the American food industry to give us healthy food that tastes good, is made from pure, life-enhancing ingredients and does not cost a fortune. These are attainable goals.

I LOVE ICE CREAM

ICE CREAM!! The mere thought of that deliciously sweet, creamy substance can actually make my mouth water and it feels almost UNAMERICAN to be critical of it in any way. However, my job is to inform and educate...so here goes (and please don't hate me)!!! Most commercial ice cream and frozen yogurt products on the market today are synthetic from start to finish and loaded with additives that are not meant for human consumption. Fat scraps rendered from slaughterhouses, such as cooked tallow, suet and lard are used instead of cream from milk because they are a cheaper alternative and have a longer freezer life. Hydrogenated oils are often used as well and the health hazards of these trans-fats have been well documented.

Ice cream manufacturers are not required by law to list the additives used in the development of their products. Analyses have shown the following:

- *Diethyl glucol*: a cheap chemical used as an emulsifier instead of eggs. Diethyl glucol is the same chemical used in anti freeze and in paint removers.

- *Aldehyde C17*: used to flavor cherry ice cream, is an inflammable liquid which is also used in anilene dyes, plastics and rubber.

- *Piperonal*: is used in place of vanilla. This is a chemical used to kill lice.

- *Ethyl acetate*: is used to give ice cream a pineapple flavor. It is also used as a cleaner for leather and textiles and its vapors have been known to cause chronic lung, liver and heart damage.

- *Butyraldehyde*: is used in nut flavored ice cream. It is one of the ingredients of rubber cement.

- *Amyl acetate*: is used for its banana flavor. It is also used as an oil paint solvent.

- *Benzyl acetate*: is used for its strawberry flavor. It is a nitrate solvent.

Does this mean you should never again enjoy ice cream? NO!!! Next time you have a craving for it, look for the words ORGANIC on the label to insure a more wholesome product. The "super premium" brands, such as Breyers All Natural, Cascade Farms Organics or most found in your neighborhood health food store are good choices.

An example of homemade ice cream excellence is Marianne's Creamery, a Santa Cruz tradition. There are far fewer ingredients listed on the nutritional label of the more expensive varieties, (which is generally a good thing), as compared to the grocery store "house brand" versions. My standard rule of thumb is, if there are more than an inch of ingredients on any product and if I can't pronounce half of them...then I don't eat it. Period. Sorbet and fruit ices can be a healthier alternative to ice cream. However, both are still high in sugar and for most people, not something to consume on a daily basis.

If weight control is a concern, try this great recipe. Peel and freeze several organic bananas. Put the frozen bananas into a juicer, such as Champion, Acme or Juiceman type machine and out comes a cool and creamy, luscious treat...straight from nature, without the garbage, chemicals or guilt!!

REDUCING
YOUR CANCER RISK

I HAVE BEEN LONG CONVINCED that the barrage of chemicals we are exposed to in our modern life takes a toll on our health. Scientists now suspect that certain compounds, known as "endocrine disrupters" or xenoestrogens, may play a major role in the development of cancer by interfering with the action of hormones in the body. Pesticides and plastics have been shown to be prime suspects. Here are a few steps to reduce your exposure:

- *Microwave only in glass, Corning Ware, or ceramic containers.* When plastic is heated, a known carcinogenic agent, dioxin, can migrate into the food. Frozen meals should be popped out of their plastic trays prior to cooking. Yogurt cartons or butter tubs should never be used in the microwave. Do not microwave with plastic wrap—instead cover your food with a glass or ceramic lid.

- *Be careful with plastic wrap.* DEHA (di-ethylhexyl adepate) and PVC (polyvinyl chloride) are both chemicals found in cling wrap and plastic containers that disrupt hormone balance. When food is heated in it, or used as a covering, the carcinogens and xenoestrogens are transferred into the food at 200–500 parts per billion. The FDA standard is less than 0.05 parts per billion. Wraps made from polyethylene—such as Glad Crystal Clear brand—does not contain these compounds.

- *Avoid buying foods wrapped in plastic.* Buy meat and fish directly from the butcher and have the food item wrapped in paper. When buying cheese, have a wedge sliced from the wheel and have the store wrap it in paper. If you do purchase plastic wrapped foods, cut off the outermost layer which came into contact with the wrap. Store leftovers in glass or ceramic containers. The goal is to use less plasticizers in everyday life. For more information, contact Toxic Coalition (206)632-1545.

- *Choose baby products wisely.* Endocrine disrupters are believed to have an even greater negative effect on developing children. In 1997, FDA chemists found that baby bottles made from polycarbonate plastic release a plasticizer called, bisphenol A, into the infant formula during sterilization. Use glass bottles (tempered glass is available) or plastic ones made from polyethylene or polypropylene, which are free of plasticizers. Avoid pacifiers, toys, or teething rings made from polyvinyl chloride. Contact Mothers and Others For A Livable Planet at (888)ECO-INFO

- *Don't use chemical pesticides.* Use natural alternatives in your home, garden or with your pets. Examples of healthy products include Neem, ryania, pyrethrum and rotenone.

- *Use nontoxic cleaners when possible.* Vinegar, baking soda, and borax are safe. Avoid hair care products listing octoxynol or nonoxynol among the ingredients.

- *Eat organic.* Choose organic produce whenever possible, particularly when shopping for out-of-season fruit.

We can all take steps against the war on cancer—begin today!

IS THERE A LINK BETWEEN DIET AND CANCER?

O NE OF THE GREATEST CONTROVERSIES that exists today concerns the effect of diet and disease. While diet is considered a contributing factor to heart disease, its role in cancer and other illnesses is still being debated. In an effort to educate the public, the USDA published the Dietary Guidelines for Americans. These recommendations were designed to alert the public to dietary changes that could improve nutritional eating and subsequently, health. These guidelines state:

1. Eat a variety of foods

2. Maintain ideal weight

3. Avoid too much fat, saturated fat and cholesterol

4. Eat foods with adequate starch and fiber

5. Avoid too much sugar

6. Avoid too much sodium

7. If you drink alcohol, do so in moderation

It's impossible to say that eating certain foods will definitely give you cancer, but research shows that people who consume a diet that is high in fat (the average American diet is 40–45% fat) are considerably more likely to develop cancer of the breast, colon, prostate or female reproductive system. While eating a lowfat diet may not protect you from cancer, it may reduce the likelihood that you will develop it.

Eating on the Run

HOW MANY MORNINGS have you flown out of the house, neglecting to eat breakfast, then had no time for lunch, so a few handfuls of yogurt-covered raisins would have to suffice?? By 4 o'clock, you'll most likely eat anything not nailed down. It is the time of the day when candy sales and vending machines see the most action…why? Because most junk food works quickly to elevate a low blood sugar level.

Planning what and when to eat is basic rule #1. "An ounce of preparation is worth a pound of weight loss." For those days when planning hasn't happened and you find yourself tired, hungry and ready to eat the kitchen sink, have a back up plan.

The following food suggestions are available in most any market, convenience store or fast food restaurant and are aimed at balancing the blood chemistry.

- 2 Tbsp. protein powder mixed with water or lowfat milk (keep a can of protein powder in your car)
- Sliced turkey, beef or chicken and a pear
- A baked potato with broccoli & cheese (Wendy's)
- Caesar salad with turkey or chicken
- Whole grain crackers and peanut butter (available at health food stores)
- A handful of almonds and a carton of plain nonfat yogurt
- Cottage cheese and an orange
- Chinese food—beef & broccoli (hold the sugar & MSG)
- Cut up veggies with dip and a deviled egg
- Roasted chicken or a can of tuna (Dave's brand is great!)
- 2 sticks of string cheese and an apple
- Hard boiled eggs and an orange
- Cream cheese and lox on a whole grain bagel
- Breakfast burrito made with eggs, beans & cheese (Taco Bell)
- Egg salad on celery, crackers or your finger!

GRANDMA'S CURE ALL

MOST OF US ARE FAMILIAR WITH THE OLD SAYING, "An apple a day keeps the doctor away." For years I can remember my dear old grandma starting off the day with a cup of hot water mixed with apple cider vinegar. She called it her "tonic" and said it was good for "whatever ailed you." My grandmother remained vigorous until her death at age 95.

The use of apple cider vinegar (ACV) was used throughout Biblical times to treat infections and wounds. Hippocrates, the Father of Medicine, prescribed vinegar for his patients back in 400 B.C., believing it to be effective in relieving conditions of acidosis, such as gout, arthritis, digestive problems and liver disorders—as well as germ fighting.

Modern research has shown that a single dose of ACV contains 93 different compounds all considered vital to good health and a balanced metabolism. These include powerful enzymes, a rich source of potassium, vitamins, minerals, essential amino acids and pectin.

DeForest Jarvis M.D., author of *Folk Medicine: A Vermont Doctor's Guide to Good Health*, writes: "Cider vinegar is conducive to the proper oxidation of blood and is one of nature's most perfect foods, especially if made from organically grown apples." Of all the home remedies Dr. Jarvis studied, none matched apple cider vinegar in treating such a wide variety of ills.

Uses of apple cider vinegar include:

- helps aid digestion and assimilation
- relieves sore throat and laryngitis
- acts as natural appetite suppressant and diuretic
- aids arthritis by flushing harmful toxins and crystals from joints, tissues and organs
- helps sinus, asthma and flu sufferers breathe easier
- soothes sunburn and maintains healthy skin
- helps maintain a youthful, vibrant body while slowing the natural aging process
- fights fatigue and insomnia
- maintains cardiovascular health

Old wives' tale? Medicinal folk lore, you ask? Countless people over the years have sworn ACV to be their "cure all" and "fountain of youth" without the benefit of empirical data or double-blind studies to prove its merit. Yet, recent findings by researchers from Arizona State University suggest the old folk remedy may very well be a powerful tool in the treatment of insulin resistance. When they tested volunteers with insulin resistance (a compromised ability of the cells to respond to signals from insulin and an underlying factor of Type II Diabetes, hypertension, obesity, and blood lipid abnormalities) who had ingested 2 tablespoons of ACV prior to a high-glycemic meal, designed to quickly drive the blood sugar up, they found the blood sugar and insulin levels of those receiving the vinegar to be significantly lower than the placebo group. Overall, there was a 37% improvement in insulin sensitivity. Interestingly, a control group without insulin resistance also demonstrated an improvement in insulin sensitivity, suggesting that ACV in some way slows down the quick blood sugar/insulin response to high-glycemic foods.

The standard recipe is 1–2 teaspoons ACV to one 8-oz. glass water daily. One can increase or decrease the amount of vinegar used and the number of cups per day, depending on taste and tolerance. For sweetness, 1–2 teaspoons of honey or stevia to taste can be added to the mixture. I add a little bit of lemon juice to my drink and prefer the water to be warm. Try it in lieu of coffee in the morning. I can hear my Granny now saying, "Try it! What have you got to lose?"

Food Facts 💜

BREAKFAST
THE MOST IMPORTANT MEAL OF THE DAY

A COMMON PROBLEM I'VE SEEN WHILE COUNSELING thousands of weight-challenged people is that most of them do not eat breakfast. Either they are not hungry first thing in the morning, they have no time or they don't like breakfast foods. For one reason or another, breakfast is eliminated and for many of these folks, perhaps twelve, fourteen, sixteen hours have gone by without any intake of food whatsoever. Then from lunch on, or more typically, from dinner and into the night, they bulk up on calories in a disproportionate window of time, resulting in,

you guessed it...FAT!

By eating breakfast, ideally within one hour of arising, the metabolism starts burning and blood sugar levels normalize, balancing the body's chemistry for a good part of the day. No other meal has as profound an effect, because typically at no other time during the day is one's body responding to the awakening state. Without a doubt, breakfast is important to eat, so get yourself into the habit. Even if the thought of morning food makes you nauseous, you'll get over it.

Personally, I do best with protein in the morning. When I eat carbohydrates for the A.M. meal, I always get sugar cravings later in the day. I have tested this a hundred times and know that by 3 or 4 P.M., look out. I must have something sweet and I can't shake it off until I do. If I eat eggs or cottage cheese or a piece of chicken from the night before—no problem!

Here are some five-minute-or-less breakfast suggestions that adhere to **The Healthy Way** weight loss program!

- *Micro Eggs:* In a coffee cup, whisk 1 to 3 eggs with a splash of nonfat milk and a dash of salt. Microwave for one minute. Grab a fork and go.

- *Breakfast Burrito:* Follow recipe above, also adding 3 Tbsp. salsa and 2 Tbsp. grated nonfat/lowfat cheddar cheese. Place a whole wheat tortilla on top of the cup or bowl as it is being microwaved. Then spoon mixture into tortilla, roll it up and away you go.

- Nonfat cottage cheese mixed with plain yogurt and 1 Tbsp. of no-sugar orange marmalade (or any flavor no sugar jam).

- 2 hard boiled eggs and an orange or apple.
- Oatmeal, flaxseeds, fruit and unsweetened soy milk—microwave for 40 seconds and it's ready.
- Just a piece of whole grain toast would be better than nothing!
- Be careful with cereal as many varieties are high in sugar and carbohydrates. Barbara's Shredded Wheat, Kashi and Keto Krisp brands are the best for weight loss.
- Make foods ahead of time that can last the whole week. Suggestions and recipes are available in the *Healthy Way Cookbook*.
- Make a tray of deviled eggs with lowfat mayo (Spectrum Naturals makes a good organic version).
- Bake up a lowfat quiche or frittata on Sunday morning and have it for breakfast for several days.
- Make a batch of whole grain waffles or pancakes and freeze in individual baggies. Then when in a hurry, place in toaster, top with lowfat/nonfat cottage cheese, nonfat yogurt or all-fruit jam.
- *Basic Breakfast Shake:*

  1 cup frozen fruit

  2 scoops low carb protein powder

  1 cup nonfat milk, unsweetened soy milk or mineral water

  handful of ice cubes

  1 tsp. vanilla extract

Place ingredients into blender and in the time it takes to put toothpaste on your toothbrush you will have a nutritious drink.

ALLERGIES AND FOOD SENSITIVITIES

NOTHING IS MORE FRUSTRATING OR CHALLENGING TO AN INDIVIDUAL who is adhering to a weight loss program than when, hard as they try, the scale just doesn't move. Another confusing situation is when inch loss exceeds weight loss. Clothes are loose and the mirror reflects a change, yet the scale doesn't show a loss.

Do not for a minute believe that all those in the overweight population are lazy and overindulgent or lie about what they eat. I have found for myself and a large number of my clients, some people's weight loss doesn't happen to the degree of others doing the same exact program, despite exercise and balanced food intake. I believe this occurs in response to allergies and food sensitivities. Many people are overweight because a significant part of their diet consists of foods that contribute to inflammation.

Physiology
When allergens, toxins, and other stressors are released, blood vessels and capillaries in the injured area dilate to enable the body's healing substances to get to the injured site quickly. At the same time, capillary walls become more permeable and fluids force their way into the surrounding tissues. The accumulated fluid and waste cause inflammation, which in turn, can result in gaining weight.

Food allergies and sensitivities often trigger an outpouring of responses which promote fluid retention, bloating and weight gain. Approximately 25 percent of the population have subclinical allergies to wheat and dairy products. Other foods that commonly trigger allergic reactions are peanuts, corn, soy, chocolate, coffee, tomatoes, bananas, oranges, wines, mushrooms, and parmesan cheese. Keep in mind that most people don't even realize they are experiencing an allergic reaction to foods because of the subtle nature of symptoms. They often crave the foods to which they are most allergic.

Determining If an Allergy Exists
To determine if you have a food allergy, start by eliminating one of the most common allergens, either wheat or dairy. Choose one. Do not do both at the same time. Completely eliminate that single food item from your diet for seven days. Check labels and be fastidious in its complete elimination.

On the morning of the eighth day, eat a full serving size of the suspected food. For example, if you are eliminating wheat, have wheat toast, cream of wheat, wheat bran muffin or wheat pasta. After ingestion, for the next four hours be aware of any reactions such as bloating, fatigue, congestion, hunger, anxiety, headaches, gastrointestinal problems, depression, confusion, etc. Again at lunch, eat a full serving of the suspected allergen for verification and watch for signs and symptoms. If there is no reaction 4 hours after lunch, one can assume this particular food is not an allergen. Next day—choose another suspected food and repeat the seven day process as outlined above.

Helpful Suggestions

1. Avoid the allergen completely! Get in the habit of reading labels and ask questions of food preparers. Be watchful of symptoms.

2. MSM (Methylsulfonylmethane) is a powerful anti-inflammatory known to reduce allergies. In a study published in the *Annals of the New York Academy of Sciences*, MSM reduced the tendency toward food allergies. Food sensitive individuals were able to eat foods they normally could not tolerate. 1000mg capsule of MSM 2–3 times a day with meals is the recommended dosage.

3. Whole ground flaxseed or flaxseed oil decreases inflammation, enhances immune function, helps relieve allergic symptoms, as well as being beneficial against all major degenerative conditions. One Tbsp. of oil or 2–5 Tbsp. of ground seed daily is the suggested amount.

4. Quercetin is a bioflavinoid of the Vitamin C family. It discourages mast cell release of histamine and other inflammatory compounds. 300–600mg, 1–2 times per day is the standard dosage. May be taken with bromelain to enhance absorption.

5. Give up sugar or significantly reduce its presence in the diet. All forms of sugar place a great demand on the pancreas and much higher levels of digestive enzymes are secreted to breakdown foods. Sugar is a vasoconstrictor, decreasing the flow of oxygen and nutrients to the cells.

THE WRINKLE CURE

D R. NICHOLAS PERRICONE, a dermatologist and Assistant Clinical Professor at Yale University School of Medicine, made a big stir on PBS television with his claims of anti-aging. His book entitled, *The Wrinkle Cure* has been on the *New York Times* Bestseller's List.

In a nutshell, his skin care regimen is based on anti-oxidant and anti-inflammatory research and includes topical applications of the following components:

- Vitamin C Esters
- Alpha Lipoic Acid
- DMAE (Dimethylaminoethanol)
- Tocotrienols (High potency Vitamin E)
- Alpha hydroxy and Beta hydroxy Acids

In addition, an entire chapter in his book is dedicated to healthy eating and is essentially the plan advocated by **The Healthy Way** since 1986! Dr. Perricone is quoted as saying "All the creams, lotions and topical potions in the world could never substitute eating the right diet." To summarize Dr. Perricone's dietary research, he believes foods which create inflammation and an unstable blood sugar level wreak havoc, not only with one's complexion, but overall health. Years of research have proven that the best diet formula to prevent everything from the visual effects of aging, to heart disease and cancer, is to eat an adequate portion of protein, choose low insulin producing complex carbohydrates and select fruits and vegetables rather than refined, processed foods.

Insulin in high levels tends to create chemicals in the body that encourage inflammation, which kick start the aging process. By eating foods that have a low insulin producing potential (known as low glycemic index) the sugar is delivered more slowly, keeping one's blood sugar level stable.

In addition, sugar interacts with the collagen of the skin—a process known as glycosylation. When sugar attaches to the protein strands of collagen, cross links occur, no longer allowing for free movement. As a result the skin becomes sagging, inflexible, wrinkly and prone to age spots.

Furthermore, excess sugar in the diet can cause the single bond of collagen's molecular chain to become double bonds. These double bonds act like magnets to free radicals, which clearly cause age acceleration and degenerative disease.

Dr. Perricone's Anti-Aging Foods and Strategies

- *Water*   8–10 glasses/day (The true fountain of youth)
- *Protein*   Up to 12–14oz/day (lots of fish), more if you are very active
- *EFA*   Use fish, flax and olive oils, raw seeds and nuts to keep a balance between Omega 3 and Omega 6 fatty acids
- *Plain Yogurt*   The *lactobacillus acidophilus* in yogurt is a probiotic; limit other dairy sources
- *Learn to graze*   Eat four to six small well-balanced meals a day to keep the insulin level balanced.
- *Stay away from high glycemic carbohydrates such as:*

breads	white pasta	all refined and processed foods
bananas	corn	white rice
cookies	candy	fruit juices
cakes	pancakes/waffles	

- *Limit red meat*
- *Beware of sugar in all its forms*

HISTORY OF
THE AMERICAN DIET

AMERICANS ARE NOW THE FATTEST PEOPLE ON THE PLANET. We try liquid drinks, prepackaged meals, shots, pills, you name it...we try it in our quest to get thin. Yet, the real problem lies in the Standard American Diet, which is S.A.D. for short. Many of the foods we eat today are not the foods our bodies were designed to use for fuel.

According to the discordance theory, in looking at our ancestors, genetically we possess the same DNA of 40,000 years ago. However, our environment, and especially our food, has radically changed. Researchers conclude that our Paleolithic ancestors were muscular and ate an average of five pounds of food per day, whereas the current American consumes an average of about three pounds per day.

Generations ago they ate what they could pick with their hands, dig from the ground or kill. Berries, nuts, fruit, vegetables, leaves, grasses, bulbs, fungi, flower shoots, roots and whatever fish or animal they could trap. Ninety nine percent of man's time on earth, we've basically eaten one way. It's only been a relatively short time period since our nutrition has been altered. We still possess Stone Age physiology that needs to contend with a 21st Century diet. The problem is, we just haven't evolved long enough.

The Industrial Revolution, just 200 years ago, brought the birth of agricultural technology and some of the most powerful events in all of human history. It has been less than 60 years since processed foods were invented. During World War II, food chemists needed a way to get large amounts of food to the troops in remote area. This lead to the advent of processed, prepackaged, dehydrated, chemically preserved foods. The first frozen meal hit the marketplace in 1949 with Swanson T.V. dinners.

Other factors that have changed the face of our nutrition include a greater number of women joining the work force and thus less home cooked meals, as well as television which has created a more sedentary lifestyle. In addition, commercial advertising has radically changed our dietary practices. In 1997, Coca Cola spent $277 million dollars on their advertising campaign (Pepsi spent $200 million). In contrast, the American Cancer Society had only $1 million to promote their "Five a Day" campaign to have Americans increase their consumption of fruits and vegetables.

John McDougal, MD, best selling author and director of St. Helena Health Center, claims half of all grocery store items are now processed and altered in some fashion. Presently, the average American consumes approximately 20 pounds of preservatives per year.

Clearly, of all the changes in the U.S. diet, sugar consumption rates the highest, increasing more than 75 times since the early 1900s. Termed the "dietary shock of the 21st century," such an enormous increase of glucose molecules bombarding one's system creates stress, especially on the pancreas. Is it any wonder why diabetes rates are skyrocketing?

The changes in the American diet have occurred in a very short time span and many authorities feel we haven't conducted this experiment long enough to witness all the ramifications. Our great nation may be the home of the free and the brave, but unfortunately we are also home to the fattest and highest consumers of processed foods. With greater awareness, these sad facts could get turned around for the better in a relatively short period of time. Why not start today by getting back to basics!

OBSERVATIONS OF A WEIGHT LOSS COUNSELOR

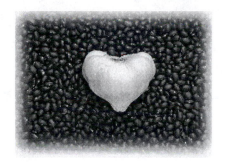

THE TRUTH

AN ENORMOUS PUBLIC HEALTH PROBLEM that exists in the U.S. is how we are fueling our bodies or lack thereof. The discussion of weight, health and nutrition in America has become so skewed with unrealistic beauty and body standards, that it's little wonder many people feel angry and uncertain. But let us not confuse the issue with our emotions. Fit, strong, full of life force and well nourished...these are the ideals we must strive for.

Being aware of what is put into our mouths is the single most effective health strategy one can take. This is also a profound declaration of self love. How we feed ourselves can be a most nurturing act. The Latin word for diet, "Diaeta," means "way of life." One day of overeating has never made anybody fat...it's the day in and day out behaviors that dictate our waist! Basically, the American diet has become one of convenience.

A true fact: by the year 2025, which isn't far off, every single American will be overweight if we keep up with the current trend. Just twenty years ago, one out of four Americans were considered overweight. Today, it's one out of two! Americans are the fattest people on the planet. "This epidemic of obesity we are faced with will cost the general public health budget hundreds of billions by 2020...making HIV look economically like a bad case of the flu!" This quote was made by William Dietz, director of nutrition at the Center for Disease Control.

We can thank fast food, video games, cuts in school exercise programs, anything "supersized," and most pre-packaged, processed foods for assisting in the deadly fattening of our youth. Obesity is up by 40% in the 12 to 15 age group.

Okay...no more doom and gloom statistics. The good news is we now have enough information on longevity and wellness to plan on living until 95–100 years old. The number of centenarians (100 year olds) doubled in the last 10 years. Now there are more than 70,000 alive today in the U.S. So some folks are doing it right. The bottom line, we as a country need to develop an "eating for health" program that aids in our quality as well as quantity of life. Health and nutrition were never meant to be this complicated.

Tips to Maximize Weight Loss

- Weigh yourself a few times a week.
- Prevent hunger by spreading food throughout the day.
- Be sure to eat; don't starve yourself.
- Temporarily omit prepackaged /processed foods.
- Keep it fresh and simple.
- Complete a food journal.
- Exercise at least 30 minutes per day. Walk up a sweat!
- Drink plenty of water each day. Eight 8-oz. glasses minimum.
- Eat on time and on schedule.
- Be prepared. Have a large salad, fresh fruit, barbecued, grilled or baked chicken or seafood on hand for quick and easy access.
- Cut back on diet drinks and coffee. These beverages can affect weight loss in sensitive individuals. Do not use flavored waters sweetened with sugar substitutes, corn syrup or fruit juices. Artificial sweeteners can make some people gain weight.
- Remember ¼ teaspoon of salt will retain ½ pound of water.
- Are you getting enough rest? Do you now, or have you recently, had a cold?
- Have a variety of things to eat. Don't stick to the same foods.
- Eat one fish meal regularly (several times a week).
- Over-the-counter medications can slow weight loss as well as prescribed drugs. Are you taking: cough drops, birth control pills, antibiotics?
- Remember, processed/packaged deli meats and poultry won't help you lose weight. Check to see if it has been injected with butter, sodium or broth! When using ground chicken or turkey, be sure to use white meat or ground breast only.
- Believe in yourself!!! You can lose weight and keep it off!!!

EXCUSES

"The cleaners shrunk my outfit."

"Just this once won't matter."

"I deserve it."

"I'll start again tomorrow."

"It doesn't matter."

"Mom will be mad if I don't eat what she cooks."

"It's genetic."

"I can't change."

"It's that time of the month."

"One bite won't hurt."

"It says fat free."

"Why even try—I've failed before and I'll fail again."

"I'm too short for my weight."

"My skin will sag if I lose weight."

"I don't have time to eat right."

"I can't offend the hostess."

"I don't know how and I can't learn."

"Can't teach an old dog new tricks."

"It's too hard."

"I'm too young."

"I'm too old."

"It's Christmas."

"It's our anniversary."

"It's Halloween."

"It's my Birthday."

"It's New Year's Eve."

"It's Ground Hog Day!"

Excuses do not get results!
Honesty Does!
Love yourself enough to commit!

OPRAH'S TOP 10

OPRAH WINFREY, the world's most famous "yo-yo" dieter, through her years of struggling, has helped many of us weight challenged folk to realize, it doesn't matter how much money or intelligence or power one has adipose tissue (also known as FAT) happens to the best of us! Oprah's previous attempts at quick weight loss schemes were painful to watch as she'd slim down, then balloon up again before our very public eyes. Now, however, it appears she's found her winning formula.

Here is her 10 point strategy:

1. Exercise 5–7 days a week
2. Exercise in the morning to boost metabolism and push yourself beyond
3. Exercise 20–60 minutes each session
4. Eat a lowfat, low sugar balanced diet
5. Eat 2 fruits and 3 vegetables each day
6. Eat 3 meals and 2 snacks each day
7. Eliminate or limit alcohol
8. Drink 6–8 glasses of water every day
9. Stop eating 2–3 hours before bedtime
10. Renew your commitment each day

Observations ❤

TESTIMONIALS

When Jean Thomas first came to **The Healthy Way**, she was using a cane for assistance. She required insulin injections for her brittle diabetes, and her tears spoke of the untold pain in being 100 plus pounds overweight. Like many others, Jean had tried literally everything to lose weight without success. Within two weeks of beginning the program, she was able to get rid of her cane. Two weeks after that, her doctor was able to take her off insulin, after 15 years of daily use! Seven weeks into the program she had lost 21 pounds and gained a new lease on life. Why?? Because she broke her addiction to sugar and finally had a stable blood sugar level.

Carlotta Wilcox another of our special clients, came to us needing to lose over 200 pounds. She was essentially homeless and through our scholarship program, successfully lost 71-½ pounds in 35 weeks. Carlotta did this without a kitchen of her own or certain conveniences many of us take for granted. If she could stick to the program and make it work, then anyone can.

Don Walker, a local hardware store owner, lost 140 pounds in seven months, an average of 4.4 pounds per week. He's maintained his weight for more than five years by following a low glycemic food plan Monday through Saturday. Then on Sunday, he eats whatever he wants, although he typically stays away from sweets. Chicken and dumplings, pasta alfredo, you name it, he eats it one day per week and then gets back to a healthier regime.

All of the counselors at our center would fight over who would get to see client *Robin Gabriel-Holden*, a beautiful woman who worked hard to lose 60 pounds and gain a whole new life. She was so happy with the program that she left her retail sales position to become a weight loss counselor at **The Healthy Way**. That was almost ten years ago and she remains a powerful example of inspiration.

Michelle Lewis, a UCSC student, struggled to lose weight. She would lose 2 pounds one week and gain 3 pounds on her next visit into the center. It took her 2 years to lose 25 pounds, but in the process she learned what her particular needs were in keeping the weight off. It's been eight years now and she is still maintaining her weight loss.

There is a feeling of joy and accomplishment in all weight loss stories. However when children succeed, the sense of reward can be even greater. Twelve-year-old *Sarah* had been known in her sixth grade class at school, as "fatty, fatty two by four." She started **The Healthy Way Program** on the last day of school and in conjunction with her supportive family, she spend her summer vacation improving her eating and exercise habits. Over the three months, Sarah lost 25 pounds and started Junior High School with a newfound sense of confidence about her figure and her self esteem.

It is such an honor and a privilege for myself and **The Healthy Way** staff to witness these incredible transformations. Everyday we see another miracle! Our mission is to assist our clients in finding peace with food, greater harmony through life sustaining habits, and freedom from negative body image issues. We believe nutrition and lifestyle are the basic fundamentals of preventive medicine. Since 1986 we have pioneered a cutting edge approach to wellness, and our outstanding long-term success speaks for itself.

Our clients consistently achieve an average weight loss of 2.5 pounds per week, as well as a 60% long term weight maintenance success rate after two years. The national average is 95% of dieters gain all their weight back within one year. When nutritional changes are incorporated into one's existing lifestyle, new habits are easier to maintain. This is the service we provide at **The Healthy Way.** We believe you don't have to know the way to be willing to go and in the end, the only people who fail are those who don't try.

If you, the reader, have maintained a weight loss achieved with the help of **The Healthy Way,** we would be most interested in speaking with you. Our phone number is (831) 462-5900.

If you have maintained a weight loss of 30 pounds or more for at least a year and would like to enter the National Weight Control Registry, a database of successful dieters compiled by the Universities of Pittsburgh and Colorado, call (800) 606-6927.

BEFORE AND AFTER PHOTOS

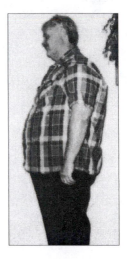

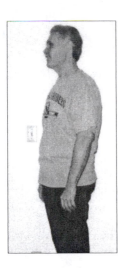

"When I was overweight, my working days were pretty much over. It was difficult for me to even move. Thanks to the support and guidance from the counselors at **The Healthy Way***, I have regained my health and my life. I have been maintaining my weight loss for the past five years. I am a new man."*

Don Walker
Felton, Ca.

Lost 140 lbs & 152 inches

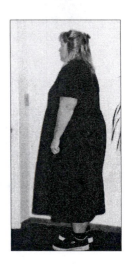

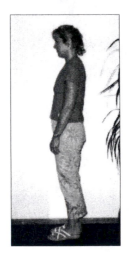

"I never realized I was capable of accomplishing something such as reaching my goal. Now I feel I have the confidence to do anything! I have maintained my weight loss within 1 to 2 pounds for over a year now. The accountability at **The Healthy Way** *makes all the difference for me!"*

Kathleen Boynton
Felton, Ca.

Lost 139.5 lbs & 166 inches

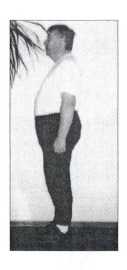

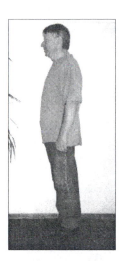

"*I whole heartedly recommend* **The Healthy Way** *program. It will change your life.*"

Harry Shippy
Capitola , Ca.

Lost 65 lbs & 67 inches

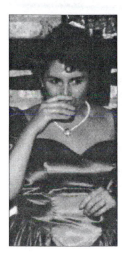

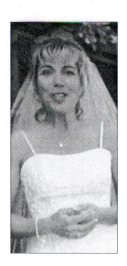

"**The Healthy Way** *helped me to transform my body, as well as my life. Through the program, I acquired life skills that I apply to aspects of my life other than weight control. I was so impressed with the program, I quit my career in retail to become a* **Healthy Way** *counselor and that was almost ten years ago!!*"

Robin Gabriel-Holden
Santa Cruz, Ca.

Lost 60 lbs & 65 inches

ONE HUNDRED YEARS OF DIETS

1898   Chewing 100 times per minute is the weight loss trend and is recommended as a digestive aid.

1918   America's first selling diet book hits the market—*Diet and Health with Key to the Calorie* by Lulu Hunt Peters.

1919   The first Health-O-Meter bathroom scale is manufactured.

1929   Advertisements encourage women to reach for a cigarette rather than a "sweet."

1930   The "Hollywood Grapefruit Diet" is the rage—585 calories a day for 18 days!

1934   Latex girdles are invented.

1942   The Metropolitan Life Insurance company publishes tables of "ideal weights" based on gender, height, and frame size.

1948   Two-thirds of patients treated for obesity are prescribed amphetamines.

1951   Jack LaLanne's first television broadcast.

1958   Saccharin comes to sweeten up life.

1961   Weight Watchers becomes established.

1963   Tab, the first diet soda, is born.

1967   Twiggy—the world's first super model—5'7" and 92 lbs.

1972   Everyone is on the Dr. Atkins Diet (High protein and fat, low carbs).

1978   Everyone is now on the Scarsdale Diet (High protein, low carbs).

1979   The Pritikin Diet is catching on as the new diet trend (high fiber, no sugar, no salt and less than 10% fat).

1980   The term "Anorexia Nervosa" first appears in the diagnostic manuals.

1981   Beverly Hills Diet—nothing but grapefruit for 10 days.

1982   First liposuction procedure is performed in the U.S.
(Today it is the #1 cosmetic procedure).

1983   Burn calories with Jane Fonda's workout video.

1988   Optifast is the rage as Oprah Winfrey loses 67 lbs. on the liquid diet.

1988   Six months later, Oprah gains all her weight back, plus some, and the failure of liquid diets becomes clear.

1995   Everyone is talking about "The Zone" (P.S. **The Healthy Way** has been offering a "zone" based diet for over 12 years now!)

1996   6 million Americans are taking Phen-Fen diet pills.

1997   Phen-Fen is banned by the FDA due to deaths and severe side effects.

1998   Xenical the newest fat blocker hits the market (and can cause a number of gastrointestinal problems including rectal leakage)!!!

If Not Now, When?

DO YOU FEEL PRESSURED that there just aren't enough hours in the day to get into shape? There is actually no better time than the present to get started on a health building regimen. After years of being both time stressed and weight challenged, I've become more healthy and have actually gained more time in my life by following a few guidelines.

Exercise: It's a must! The benefits have been documented and could fill an entire library. Set "do-able" goals for an exercise plan, one you can stick with and one you enjoy doing. Join a gym, dance around your house, go up and down the stairs a dozen times or take your dog for a walk. It's good to sweat. Exercise first thing in the morning ensures that it gets done and is out of the way. Energy is motion. Nothing will give you more energy or improve your attitude better than moving your body. Researchers confirm that the total accumulation of exercise in a 24 hour period is what counts, so even short intermittently spaced bouts of exercise offer great benefits. But if you have any health problems, be sure to contact your physician before embarking upon any exercise program.

Get On a Food Plan: Diet has become such a four letter word, so let's call it an "eating for health" regime. You're choosing, not cheating. Without balance, without some type of structure, most folks will succumb to weight gain. One's diet should be looked at on an individual basis. There are many physiological, as well as psychological factors that can interfere with a successful eating strategy. Once I cleaned up my diet and limited the things that didn't work well in my body—both my weight and stress level decreased.

Support: There is nothing as constant as change, and few things in life are as challenging as making a change. Research has proven the benefits of a supportive environment, either individually or in a group setting. People often need help achieving mastery over a habit or addiction. It's hard work to quiet that inner judge or critic. By learning to listen to the inner ally, that friend within each of us can be better heard.

Clinical Guidance: The Phen-fen diet pill fiasco has had some tragic side effects. Yet people are hungry for a dietary aid that can curb the appetite. I've found several supplements such as B complex, 5-hydroxytryptophan, MSM, and St. John's Wort to be helpful for those people requiring additional support. These substances are generally far safer than anything a pharmaceutical company has to offer.

On those occasions when you have overeaten, be sure to drink more water and exercise longer than your normal routine the next day. Get back to your program. Don't overeat two days in a row.

BENEFITS OF JOURNALING

I N THE FIELD OF HEALTH AND WEIGHT LOSS, there is rarely a consensus among industry professionals, as beliefs and opinions vary greatly. However, one practice everyone agrees upon is keeping a food journal. By doing so, one can gain greater insight and mastery over their body and emotions.

The initial response to a food diary is met with moans, groans and "Do I have to?" In all my years of practice, I've yet to meet someone who didn't derive benefit from doing so and in a short time, they realize the positive aspects as well.

Journaling helps to keep us honest. By writing down everything that goes into our mouths, our attention and focus as to what, when and why we eat, becomes more clear. Patterns, such as infrequency of eating or late night snacking can be observed and strategized.

Studies on the topic of unconscious eating state that we may inadvertently consume 1,000 extra calories per day without realizing we are doing so. Research has shown that 80% of us—even lean, athletic people—underestimate their food intake and overestimate consumption of healthier items, such as fruits and vegetables. Journaling gives us the opportunity to pay closer attention.

Food allergies and intolerances can also reveal themselves with the aid of a food diary by correlating symptoms with dietary intake of a suspected allergen.

Another benefit of journaling is that it helps us see the connection between food and the body/mind. What we eat or don't eat has an enormous effect on our mood, energy level and mental outlook. Journaling brings into focus, behaviors and thought patterns that may not be conducive to health and/or established goals.

Like a private diary, journaling lets us be alone with our thoughts and feelings. We can make greater personal discoveries when freed from the constraints of judgements and social scrutiny. Without shame or guilt, reasons such as why the whole bag of cookies needed to be eaten can reveal themselves when the journal is used for private, independent exploration.

It is also an opportunity to nurture ourselves, to note accomplishments and give strokes. Just keeping the journal in itself feels constructive and positive.

Rachel Naomi Ramen, MD, bestselling author and a long time counselor to cancer patients, finds that life's meaning can become more clear when asking ourselves the following three questions and writing down the answers.

They include:

What surprised me today (this week or this month)

What touched or moved me

What inspired me

There is no right or wrong way to keep a food journal. Some people write in it after every meal, others wait until the end of the day to note what was eaten. Some folks prefer to write down what they will eat the day before and will then adhere to the prepared menu by checking off in the journal what has been consumed.

In regards to weight loss, the counseling staff at **The Healthy Way** states without question that the most effective technique for greater fat loss is keeping an accurate food journal. The process of writing down what has been eaten makes one accountable, aware and a much more successful dieter. The added benefit of "aversion therapy", not wanting to write down "one pint Häagen-Dazs ice cream and six Mint Milano cookies" often helps the individual not to partake in the activity.

See the following two pages for examples of easy-to-follow journal formats we advocate at **The Healthy Way.**

"The secret of success is to go from one failure after another without loss of enthusiasm." ~Winston Churchill

Date	Food Eaten	Protein	Starch	Vegetable	Fruit	Oil	Feelings/Comments
Breakfast							
Snack							
Lunch							
Snack							
Dinner							
Snack							

Water ▢▢▢▢▢▢▢   Supplements ▢▢▢▢▢▢▢   Vitamin A.M. ▢ P.M. ▢   Exercise:

What happened today? (Big and small achievements, obstacles, pitfalls, discoveries, frustrations, slips, victories, etc.)

"Never let a day go by without giving at least three people a compliment. Begin with yourself." ~ **The Healthy Way**

Date	Protein	Starch	Vegetable	Fruit	Oil	Hunger Level	Where?	Emotion
Breakfast								
Snack								
Lunch								
Snack								
Dinner								
Snack								
Water ▢▢▢▢▢▢	**Supplements** ▢▢▢▢▢▢		**Vitamin A.M.** ▢ **P.M.** ▢			**Exercise:**		

What happened today? (Big and small achievements, obstacles, pitfalls, discoveries, frustrations, slips, victories, etc.)

LATE NIGHT EATING

C AN EATING AT NIGHT AFFECT ONE'S WEIGHT? Those late meals may indeed be responsible for weight gain. Given the busy schedules most of us keep where we juggle kids, odd work hours and overtime at the office, dinner is often put on a back burner and takes place late in the evening. Researchers have found that people who eat late tend to consume more calories than those who don't. Most obese individuals they studied consumed more than half their total daily calories after 6 P.M. The problem with eating late is you're stockpiling fuel for the least active part of your day, the hours that you sleep. Instead of being burned up as fuel, the food you eat before bed has more of a chance of being stored as fat.

Joseph Kasof, Ph.D., a specialist in social behavior at the University of California at Irvine, concludes that light can affect how much people eat and found that the less light there was, even to a small degree, would cause people to overeat. His suggestion is to turn the lights up when eating.

Granted, if you exercise frequently or have a high-revving metabolism, nocturnal noshing isn't that big a deal. But if you spend most of your days confined to a desk only to come home and ride the couch, late night eating will typically cause weight gain.

There is an extreme form of late night eating, known as "night eating syndrome", in which those afflicted eat nothing or very little during the day and then consume 50–100% of their daily calories after dinner hours, often waking up in the middle of the night to eat. Albert Stunkard, MD., a psychiatrist who first identified the disorder, estimates at least 5% of the U.S. population suffers from the disorder. The syndrome tends to be precipitated by stress and becomes a chronic, habitual problem over time. Typically the late night snacks are high in carbohydrates, which raise the levels of serotonin in the brain, helping people to relax and sleep.

For many of us, eating earlier is just impossible, so what can be done to minimize the consequences of a late night eating schedule? Try these steps:

- Schedule snack times throughout the day. Eating a big dinner causes the body to produce excess insulin, a hormone that can cause fat storage. Consuming a series of smaller meals throughout the day helps to keep insulin levels low, meaning you'll burn calories more efficiently, even at night.

- Eat your largest meals in the morning and afternoon. Consume most of your calories before 3 P.M. You will be fueling yourself for the most active part of the day.

- Exercise! Research indicates that exercise suppresses the appetite, so you'll be less likely to exceed the feed limit. Take a few minutes out for a light jog, a series of jumping jacks or some sit-ups before or after dinner.

- A good rule of thumb is to stop eating 2–3 hours prior to bedtime which allows for proper digestion.

- Don't skip breakfast or lunch. The best way to reduce overeating at night is to eat adequately during the day.

- Eating a hearty snack at 4 or 5 P.M. will help you to have less of an appetite at dinner time and prevent overeating.

VACATION EATING

O N HOLIDAY, WHO WANTS TO MONITOR EVERY FORKFUL? No one! That's why the typical vacationer gains weight. Many people abandon all rules of healthy eating while on vacation. But too much calorie-laden, fatty food can ruin a holiday because it can lead to unwanted weight gain, feelings of guilt and can zap the energy you need to enjoy sight-seeing activities.

These tips can help you begin to identify high risk situations and to help plan alternative behaviors:

- When traveling by air, don't leave yourself at the mercy of airport food. Pack healthy snacks in your carry-on bag. Fresh fruit and vegetables, low carb protein bars; lowfat, high fiber, low carb crackers such as RyVita or Finn Crisp.

- Bring along books, stationary or hobbies you can work on to keep yourself occupied during layovers.

- Request a lowfat meal when you book your airline ticket. Better yet, order a "diabetic meal" and you will receive more fresh and natural foods.

- When traveling by car, plan occasional stops so you can stretch and walk. Pack plenty of healthy snacks (such as those described for air travel) and a jug of water.

- Make exercise an integral part of your vacation plans. Pack your walking shoes and use the hotel swimming pool or fitness center.

- Drink water! It's easy to confuse thirst for hunger when it's humid.

- Skip the "free" breakfast offered at many hotels/motels which often consists of Danish, doughnuts and muffins. Instead, select fruit, scrambled eggs or oatmeal.

- Watch the alcohol, especially the "umbrella kind." Tropical cocktails typically contain rich coconut milk and sugary syrups that can add up to 400–500 calories per drink.

- Splurge, but not at every meal. The "I'll diet when I get home" mind-set can lead you from a buffet breakfast, to a three-course lunch, to a six-course dinner, after dinner drinks and what the heck, "let's have dessert too." While on vacation wait a day or two before overindulging. Mentally designate one meal as special (or a few) and go easy on the others.

- Most of all, don't forget…Vacation means going away to relax, sightsee, visit friends, shop, reduce stress…lots of activities to stimulate the senses.

TIPS FOR HEALTH

A FTER YEARS OF WORKING IN THE FIELD OF NUTRITION AND WELLNESS, I have observed that most people need to remember these simple and powerful tips:

1. *Remember to EAT!* So many folks starve themselves all day, and then by 4 P.M.—look out where are the sweets?! You can't drive without fuel and the same thing goes for your body. Eat something for breakfast—it's so important. Have lunch, dinner and maybe two fruit snacks in between. Stop eating 2–3 hours before bed. Eat foods that give to the body, rather than those which take from our systems.

2. *Drink water!* Before you reach for another diet soda or cup of coffee, make sure you've had a few glasses of water. When the body gets enough water, weight loss can increase by decreasing fluid retention, metabolizing fats from the liver, improving glandular functions and curtailing hunger.

3. *Exercise.* Find something you enjoy and just do it! To boost metabolism, exercise 5 days per week for 20–60 minutes a session. Sweating is a good thing!

4. *Make wise choices.* Eat for energy, strength and clarity. That means 80%–90% of the time, steer clear of white flour, sugar, additives and hydrogenated products. If the ingredient list is an inch or so long and you can't pronounce half the words, don't eat it! There are numerous reasons why one should shop natural and organic.

5. *Keep the faith.* Working to have a trimmer body does not mean a lifelong sentence of deprivation. Once basic metabolic functions have rebalanced themselves and desired weight has been maintained for several months, one can have overeating days without losing weight control. Having the body you want means knowing what it takes for you personally to maintain your weight, so that it becomes automatic and instinctive.

FLUID RETENTION

D O YOU FEEL BLOATED THE DAY AFTER EATING A BIG CHINESE MEAL
or perhaps the morning after having an alcoholic beverage or two? If so,
you're probably suffering from water retention (edema), a buildup of
bodily fluids in tissues that results in swelling. Menstruation, birth control pills,
and allergies can all cause water retention.

Although the precise physiological mechanism that causes edema isn't under-
stood, experts know that certain circumstances, such as eating high-sodium
foods and standing or sitting too long, can cause fluids to accumulate in the
body. Certain common medications, such as steroids, can also promote fluid
retention.

Many premenopausal women experience bloating right before their periods.
Why? According to Donald Rubell, MD, the accepted theory is that higher
ratios of estrogen to progesterone cause the body to store salt, which in turn
leads to water retention.

If you're plagued with frequent, uncomfortable bouts of edema, see a doctor.
In rare instances, bloating can signal an underlying illness such as heart or other
disorders.

- Avoid high-sodium foods. Keep your foods basic and simple. Pre-packaged,
  processed food items are notorious for salt.
- Diuretics (water pills) are not the answer. Initially they may ease water
  retention, but if taken for a long time, or in high dosages, they can have
  dangerous side effects, including dizziness, nausea, electrolyte distur-
  bances, even lung and kidney failure.
- Be sure to put your feet and legs up every chance you get.
- Lemon, B6 and apple cider vinegar are all natural diuretics. Add them to
  your water and to foods often.
- Wear support hose and steer clear of tight-fitting knee-high stocking that
  cut off the circulation.

Meals on Wheels

AMERICANS NOW EAT ONE QUARTER OF THEIR MEALS inside their cars. Our multi-tasking, no-time-to-eat lifestyle has caused the kitchen table of yesteryear to be replaced by the car dashboard, and the phenomenon is on the rise.

Ever willing to meet the changing trends, American businesses such as fast food outlets have developed laptop place mats to prevent clothes from getting soiled. Automakers such as Volvo have developed cars with refrigerated glove boxes and some models of Honda provide a pop-up table in the console. Typically, food consumed in vehicles is of a less nutritious, processed nature and is generally eaten faster than meals consumed at home or in restaurants. Our meals weren't always eaten alone or on the fly. Fact is, our ancestors spent most of their day hunting, gathering and preparing food…it was basic survival. When it came time to eat, they would do so in clans or tribes with an atmosphere of celebration. As babies, we were held while given milk and spoon feed by our caregivers. Indeed, connecting with others through food offers strong, nurturing social ties and is an integral part of our heritage. Psychologist and researcher Jeanne Achterberg summarized the importance between social support and health as follows: "Lack of social relationships constitutes a major risk factor in health, one that is even greater than smoking and appears to be a strong predictor of longevity and mortality."

Research has also shown that children of families who sit down and share a meal together have less delinquent behavior and are better students.

Without question, the busy demands of home, family and career make for challenging times. Here are a few suggestions for integrating more wholesome foods and greater social contact into your life.

1. Develop the habit of a family sabbath. Plan one meal a week (or more often) that will be home cooked amongst family and friends. Share the stories of the day.

2. Organize colleagues at work to participate in a weekly (or more often) potluck for lunch. Someone brings a salad, another brings sandwiches, pasta, whatever. Make it fun and set the precedence of healthy, yet tasty foods.

3. Brown bag it with friends once in awhile, rather than relying on fast food at meal time.

4. Investigate local restaurants and delis near work and on your route home that offer healthier cuisine. A chicken Caesar salad, Greek salad or bowl of soup to go is a far wiser choice than greasy fries, burger and milk shake.

5. If you must eat in the car…don't drive! Pull over where the atmosphere and view are pleasant (the beach, trees, kids at play). Turn off the pager and cell phone and turn on nice, relaxing music. Take ten or fifteen minutes to nourish your body.

Fat Is a
Physiological Disorder

A FEW DAYS AGO, I STOOD IN FRONT OF THE LOCAL VIDEO STORE, surrounded by a mountain of girl scout cookies as my daughter's troop sold their infamous treats. It was there, amongst the "Thin Mints" and "DoSiDos" that I was reminded of a fact I already knew. Overweight people are not gluttons or weak-willed. They do not eat more than others, and often times actually eat less! After nearly 20 years as a nutrition counselor, and also one who has personally suffered from weight issues, I am here to say that obesity is primarily a physiological disorder. Surely there is a psychological component, but we can often ask, which came first, the chicken or the egg?

Most of us want to eat cookies or some gooey treat...but the truth is, many of us can't, and just need to say no! Similar to alcoholism, those who suffer with sugar sensitivity have a difficult time practicing moderation. When they do indulge, they pay the price with added weight and/or a health problem. Any sugar addict will tell you once they give in to sweet goodies, the craving for more and more is hard to kick. It doesn't have to be about deprivation; just substitution. With the wide selection of fresh fruit available year round and all the healthy, yet tasty sugar-free options found in most stores, it's easier than ever to satisfy a sweet tooth.

Again, weight challenged people also need to be more prepared with food. Just like carrying around a baby's diaper bag with a bottle, clean diapers and a change of clothes, I encourage my clients to have apples, oranges, whole grain crackers, cans of tuna and bottled water stored in their cars. Low carb protein bars can be carried in a pocket or purse. Plan what you will eat and where you will get it.

Yes...it takes more work! Yes...it does require more energy! And right you are...it isn't fair! But each of us in life has some difficult issue (or issues) to deal with, some Achilles tendon to perhaps remind us of our humanness. On the larger scheme of things, I'm sure someone in Afghanistan or Bosnia would gladly trade problems with the weight challenged.

It seems apparent that most overweight people do not break down their carbohydrates and fats the same way thin people do. Maybe it's genetics or a sensitivity that develops from some internal factors. This we do know, blood sugar and insulin levels fluctuate greater with obesity, which stimulates the enzyme, lipoprotein lipase, known to promote fat storage. This enzyme is activated not only by high fat/high sugar/high glycemic foods, but also low calorie diets (800 calories or below), irregular eating patterns (fasting/feasting), pregnancy and hormonal shifts. Lipoprotein lipase pulls extra fat into the cells, allowing for easy storage, that is difficult to lose. In contrast, hormone sensitive lipase counteracts lipoprotein lipase by pulling fat from the cells and assisting the fat to exit the body. To date, the only thing known to stimulate this response of fat breakdown is aerobic and weight resistance exercise.

Obesity is a documented health hazard, and for most, a physical/psychological prison. Being healthy requires a responsibility to remain conscious of (cognitive, connected to, aware of, mentally registering) what goes into our mouths. Occasionally we can "unconsciously nosh", let our guard down, eat freely and not suffer the repercussions, but the operative word here is occasionally and it's different for everyone. Each of us needs to learn how far we can go and still get away with it.

Speaking for myself, it's been a lot of trial and error to finally feel good in my skin. I challenge myself by not eating certain foods which have an adverse effect on my body. Candy and junk foods go directly to my hips, cause my skin to look dull and my digestion to suffer. Focusing on being strong and healthy has helped me to evolve as a person. I believe what one eats (or doesn't eat) is the first level toward elevating consciousness. I've yet to meet an individual, fat or thin, who was clear as to their higher purpose in life while stuffing themselves with junk food.

The reason for eating a healthy, balanced diet the majority of the time is so that we might each be more present, conscious and physically fit to experience this gift of life we've been given for however long it's available to us.

HEALTHY KIDS

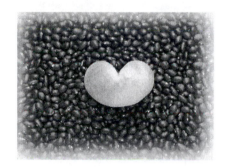

BACK TO SCHOOL LUNCHES

BACK IN THE 60s WHEN I WAS GROWING UP, nutrition and the benefits of healthy foods were not as well defined as they are today. Take, for instance, the typical brown bag lunch my mother packed me for school: a salami sandwich on white bread smothered in mayo and mustard, a bag of corn chips that left oil stains on the napkin, a can of grape or orange soda pop and a "twinkie" or "ding dong." Today, parents have much greater knowledge and a wide variety of options in providing nutritious foods for their youngsters. Here are some suggestions for packing a power lunch:

- It's best to bring lunch from home. School cafeteria menus are generally not as fresh or as healthy as those prepared at home. Try to make lunch the night before and enlist the help of your child, so that some time and forethought can go into it.

- Sandwiches made from whole grain type breads or pita pockets are more nutritious

- Peanut butter without sugar and hydrogenated fats (Adams 100% natural, Maranatha Organic or Rejuvenative Foods are good choices)

- Jam that is 100% fruit (Kozlowski Farms is tasty)

- Good old fashioned hard boiled eggs with a small packet of salt and pepper are a great source of protein.

- Carrots and celery—many come in lunch box ready packages with lowfat ranch dip already included (Earthbound Farms organics is one such company).

- Organic, 100% fruit roll-ups. Be sure it's all fruit. Some of the brands have so much sugar and chemical processing, they are equivalent to a candy bar (Cool Fruits and Fruit Leather brands are great).

- Boxed fruit juice—Be sure it says 100% juice (Hansens, Juicy Juice and Santa Cruz Organics are examples)

- Popcorn—"Ya-Ya" organic brand is great and comes in different flavors.

- Olives—black or green. Organic is always recommended.

- Yogurt—Try Brown Cow Organic whole milk for a real treat.

- Get creative! Pack up left over pasta, soup, oatmeal or potatoes…heat in the morning and put in a wide mouth thermos. The food is still warm by noon.

- Don't forget breakfast! It's a fact that kids who eat breakfast average one letter grade higher in math than do non or infrequent breakfast eaters.

FEED YOUR KIDS WELL

"TRAIN UP A CHILD in the way he should go and when he is old, he will not depart from it." With this Proverb's verse in mind, imagine how much easier it would be to change one's diet and eating habits at the age of 6 instead of 60! Today, the typical 10 year old in this country is now ten pounds heavier than a decade ago. Elevated cholesterol levels, diabetes and hypertension are more prevalent in today's youth. As we begin the new millennium, we, the caregivers of the next generation, must wake up to what goes into the tummies of our young.

A recent study that compared the USDA recommendations for kids against the results of a national polling group found that, in the real world, kids eat more junk food (fats and sweets) than meat. They eat an adequate amount of grains, but most are in the form of Spaghettios and Gold Fish crackers, rather than whole grains such as oatmeal or shredded wheat. The findings showed only 16% of children eat the recommended 3 servings of vegetables per day and that fruit was typically consumed in concentrated fruit juice form, rather than benefitting from the fiber content of whole fruit. Sad to say, soft drinks, also known as liquid candy, have surpassed water and milk as the beverage of choice.

Our children are being turned into sugar addicts without most of us even realizing it. Take attention deficit disorder (ADD) for example. According to renowned pediatric nutritionist, Fred Pescatore, M.D., today more than one third of school-aged kids line up to take their medicine for ADD. Conventional medicine sees it as a Ritalin deficiency. Drugging our children should be the absolute last resort! Hyperactivity is often the result of wild fluctuations in blood sugar levels (induced by sugar), as well as reactions to food additives, chemicals and commercial processing.

Dr. Pescatore's research shows that one teaspoon of sugar lowers the body's immune response by 50%. Mary Poppins forgot to tell us this fact when she sang "A spoonful of sugar helps the medicine go down." With the average American teen consuming 33 teaspoons of sugar per day, it is little wonder why today's kids are not as healthy as previous generations.

What's a parent to do??? Begin by learning to read food labels and discover all the hidden ingredients. Limit your child's sugar intake. The foremost way to do this is to stop having soda in the house. Offer lowfat milk, water, or watered down juice with meals. Purchase less processed foods and have more of the "real stuff" available...like chilled fruit, more whole grain breads, and crackers. Don't make fast foods be a staple, but more of a once in a while eating option. Rather than stopping at the fast food drive-thru for a kid's meal, run into the store and grab fresh apples, cheddar cheese slices, roasted turkey, olives, baby carrots and have a picnic!

Ensure a lifetime of good health for our little ones...it's the best legacy we can leave them!

Healthy Kids ❤

OVERWEIGHT KIDS

THE INCIDENCE OF OBESITY among America's youth is increasing at an alarming rate. The number of young people, ages 6–11, who are clinically defined as obese has increased by 54% since the mid 1960s. Among adolescents, ages 12–17, a 39% increase in the number has occurred in just the past ten years.

The reasons for this unprecedented rise in the number of overweight young people are simple: a poorly balanced, chemically processed diet coupled with a physically inactive lifestyle. And the sad truth is that in the vast majority of cases, overweight young people become overweight adults. In a recent journal of the American Academy of Pediatrics researchers found that girls as young as five years old experienced low self esteem when parents worry about their weight and restrict certain foods. Kids can feel bad about themselves when they eat more than they are allowed to have (the whole bag of cookies instead of a few, for instance). Restricting access to a cupboard of tempting treats is a great way to create a "sneak eater" making the forbidden food all the more desirable. Current research indicates that parent's habits, not their genetics, have the greatest influence whether a child becomes overweight. Frequently, parents have their own struggle with good eating and can make improving the diet a family project that everyone works on together.

Here are a few suggestions:

- Don't buy food items that are "off limits." Keep only healthy foods in the house so that restriction of food isn't a common concern.

- Opt for a more whole grain, less sweetened breakfast cereal. Try oatmeal or shredded wheat with raisins. Barbara's "Fruity Punch" or "Cocoa Crunch Stars" cereals, are also good and available at all health food stores. Serve with nonfat or lowfat organic milk or soy milk.

- Soda pop is the leading source of sugar in kid's diets. "Nutra Sweet" artificial sweetener should not be consumed by children due to detrimental health effects. Have water more accessible. Look for juices that are 100% juice. Juice can also be watered down. A soda on the market today called "After the Fall" spritzer is made with LoHan fruit extract and only has ten calories, 2 grams of sugar and no sodium per can. It's tasty too!

- Make protein shake smoothies as special treats. Frozen bananas placed in a juicer or food processor make a great ice cream substitute.

- Avoid fad diets, deprivation and/or criticism, as they only add to the problem. Try not to become your child's "food police."

- Make meals a special time where the whole family can sit down, relax and share the day's events.

- Turn the TV or computer off at meal time and sit at a table when eating. Watch the "mindless grazing."

- Avoid "Lunchables" and cut down on all processed foods, including fast food. Get a thermos and send pasta or soup to school. Have skimmed milk string cheese on hand. Plain nonfat yogurt with all fruit jam mixed in keeps sugar and calories down. Cottage cheese and fruit also work well for lunch, as do hard boiled eggs.

- Do physical activities with your kids and get them into sports programs. Ride your bikes together, play a game of basketball or a game of tag. The goal is to get your child moving.

- Don't reward kids with candy. Offer a trip to the movies, a backrub or a small toy as a prize for good behavior.

- Once or twice a week have an "anything goes" meal, so that deprivation doesn't become a common complaint. The child will know on Sunday, for instance, that they can have ice cream. The rest of the time, make them watered down fruit juice frozen popsicles in ice trays and let them eat as many as they want.

KIDS AND FOOD

O N A RECENT TRIP TO THE ZOO WITH MY DAUGHTER, it was interesting to read a large sign posted near the snack bar vending machines which stated, "Do not feed this food to the animals. They may get sick and die." The zoo veterinarians know very well that processed foods can endanger the health of animals-even 400 lb. gorillas, yet for many children, junk food is a mainstay in their diets.

Dr. Lendon Smith, a pediatrician and author of over 40 children's books, has stated that kids' immune systems are now half as strong as a decade ago, due in part to poor nutrition and the chemicals, preservatives, sugars, processing and additives being used. The overprescribing of antibiotics was also cited as a factor.

Today's youth have a 30–50% increase in obesity. We can look to fast foods, P.E. programs being cut in our schools, video games and our hectic "eat and run" lifestyle as the major culprits. In addition, kid's blood pressure and cholesterol levels are way up. Even more alarming, children are no longer victim to just juvenile diabetes, where they are born with a pancreatic/insulin defect. Now they are also prone to develop Type II or adult onset diabetes, where the pancreas becomes ineffective due to overuse.

There is good news, though. Evidence shows a significant improvement in the health, behavior and learning ability of our children by a strong nutritional program. What are some beginning steps toward enhancing our kids' diets? Number one is to read the label, not just the percentages, but the actual ingredients. To me, nothing represents more of a polluted kid product than "Lunchables" by Oscar Mayer. Not only is the ingredient list about two inches long, mostly with words you'd find difficult to pronounce, but the salt content (1410mg), and fat grams (18 g.) in one small serving make for a product I wouldn't feed my dog!

Sugar is another area of major concern. As stated previously, the typical American child consumes an average of 125 to 175 lbs. of sugar per year, frequently ingesting more than their own body weight. The problem with sugar is that it robs the body of important nutrients.

Soft drinks contribute the most sugar, with an average of 10 tsp. in each serving. It is alarming that many of the nation's schools have soft drink vending machines and fast food franchises right on campus, and often the proceeds fund vital school programs.

Water is the elixir of life. Make drinking water more accessible and more fun. Put it into a squeeze or sipper bottle, add fresh lemon or mint to it, serve it over ice and add a straw. Do not let kids eat NutraSweet or artificial sweeteners. The chemicals in these products have no place in a child's body and the documentation is more than conclusive. Most importantly, talk to your kids about the role nutrition plays in their lives and involve them in the process.

Internet Resource Sites for further information on children's nutrition:

www.health.gov/dietaryguidelines
www.cspinet.org/kids/index.html
www.kidshealth.org
www.niddk.nih.gov/health/nutrit/pubs/helpchld.htm

BODY IMAGE

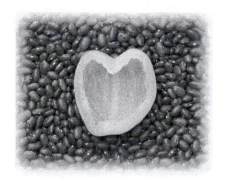

THE GREATEST GIFT
OF ALL

I JUST READ ABOUT A WOMAN IN NEBRASKA who planned to marry herself this week before 200 friends and relatives, in celebration of the fact that she is "happy with herself." I say, what a great idea! In the 12 years I've counseled people, the bottom line of what I hear being said is, "I'm not good enough," " I don't deserve..." or some variation of the same.

Self acceptance truly is a process. It appears we start out not liking ourselves as kids. Then "some things" happen to erode our sense of self, and we spend years trying to regain what we've lost. It's the game of life and all of us are players. For those challenged by weight and body image issues, this inner struggle can be even greater. Here are a few exercises that are meant to build self-esteem:

Change your vocabulary.
If you say something often enough—you'll eventually believe it. A "fat butt" can just as easily be called a "generous backside!" Try this, "I'm not overweight—I'm built for love!"

Face yourself and call a truce.
Look into the mirror, eyeball to eyeball and say a positive acknowledgment to yourself. Mirror work can be very powerful. Go ahead and tell yourself, "I love you!"

Get Strong!
Physical fitness enhances body image. Even when real deficits exist, exercise makes them easier to accept.

Accept a compliment.
No need to deny or doubt yourself. Just say, "thank you" and leave it at that.

Take a break from negative factors.
Stay away from people or situations that don't make you feel good. Don't read, watch or listen to any news for a day and see how you feel.

Give your body a voice.
How does your body feel about being "hated"? What would those body parts say to you if they could speak? Some people's tummies and thighs have never heard an encouraging word in their entire life. Send them some love and good energy.

AWAKENING TO HEALTH

I N A RECENT SURVEY OF GIRLS 13 TO 16 YEARS OF AGE, when asked what was their greatest fear, being fat rated number one, a fear greater than loss of both parents and nuclear holocaust!

In 1995, the University of Arizona studied the body satisfaction of adolescent, Caucasian females and found 90% did not like their bodies, citing perfection as 5'7" and 100 to 110 pounds.

An estimated 15 to 25% of all college age girls suffer from some type of eating disorder, be it anorexia, bulimia, compulsive overeating or binging. Males are now experiencing an increased incidence as well.

An even greater number of young people deal with a distorted body image and poor self esteem, which have crippling affects on our youth or a person of any age for that matter.

We live in a time of unprecedented extremes, where at one end of the spectrum we have individuals literally killing themselves from starvation in pursuit of thinness, while on the other, our country is now faced with an escalating epidemic of obesity, where one in three Americans are overweight. How does one make sense of such contradiction?

I believe we must wake up, become more conscious beings and strive toward *balance*. There truly is a happy medium. It's called awakening to health and requires one to be alert and attentive toward themselves.

Most eating is an unconscious act. It's a mindless, habitual, conditioned response to a number of stimuli...few of which are related to hunger.

The foremost psychological component or central core I've seen over the years, whether the client is heavy or thin is a belief that they "are not good enough," "they don't deserve" or some variation of the same.

Humans have on average, 60,000 thoughts per day. How many criticize? The only way toward balance and quieting the inner critic is to first become aware of self attacking, then establish an equal time rule, where a personal compliment must follow every criticism.

We must tend to the garden of our minds. Pull out the weeds, those useless critical attacks, and plant flower seeds...let good thoughts grow. Put the weapons down, stop the war and call a cease fire with your body and mind. It's a process, and it won't happen overnight, but it's where the focus needs to be.

Here are some "feel good about yourself" rules to implement:

- **Be nice to yourself in ways other than food.** A manicure, pedicure, massage, any type of body work is usually nurturing. Treat yourself to a workshop or retreat. Do something that makes you feel alive.

- **Keep a body image journal,** where you list the event, your belief and your response. Example: *Event*—Trying on bathing suits. *Belief*—"Nothing looks good on me." *Response*—Eat ice cream to feel better. By keeping a body image journal, your awareness to destructive patterns will be brought to light, and over time behaviors can change.

- **Celebrate diversity!** How boring if we all looked the same. Stop the body bashing and when your friends get into the cycle of it, don't participate. Appreciate all the many wonderful qualities you do possess.

- **Decrease requests for reassurance.** The more often you ask "Do I look OK?" "Do I look fat?" the more insecure you will feel. Appearance preoccupied rituals include: constantly weighing self, checking self out in every mirror, compulsively comparing self to others.

- **Get intimate with your body.** Seek out sensual experiences. Standing naked in front of the mirror stating a positive self declaration can start the body healing process. As kids our parent's looked us in the eyes with one finger shaking and scolding us. Now we do it to ourselves. You don't have to!

- **Hike, bike, go to the gym.** Work at loving your body like it's a job.

- **Do not allow others to tease or call you names.** I was referred to as "Chubs-a-buns" for more years than I care to remember.

Being fit, strong, full of life force and well-nourished...these are the ideals we must strive for.

Putting Things
in Perspective

Fact: The original sex goddess, Marilyn Monroe, had weight fluctuations between 117 and 140 pounds.

Fact: The average American woman weighs 144 lbs. and wears between a size 12–14.

Fact: Fashion models twenty years ago weighed 8% less than the average woman. Today's super models weigh 23% less.

Fact: If Barbie were a real woman, she would have to walk on all fours due to her proportions...which measure up to something like 48–10–22!

Fact: 95% of all fashion models have undergone some kind of plastic surgery.

Fact: If store mannequins were real women, they would be too thin to menstruate.

Fact: There are 3 billion women who don't look like super models and only a handful who do.

Fact: Of the handful of super models, even they don't look as good as they appear...most photography is airbrushed.

Fact: A 1995 psychological study found that three minutes spent looking at a fashion magazine caused 70% of women to feel depressed and shameful about their bodies.

It's unfortunate that we live in a time when our beauty and body standards are not based on reality. The truth is healthy, strong, and in proportion is what makes us look our best. So, turn off the T.V., put down the woman's magazine (and the "Victoria's Secret Catalog") and head for the gym or beach to do some "body watching." There you will see how wonderfully diverse all of our shapes, sizes and physical features truly are. It's time the standard we measure ourselves by, be our own.

MORE ON PERSPECTIVES

THE ARTICLE ENTITLED, "Putting Things in Perspective," which illustrates how many of our perceptions about beauty and body norms are not based on reality, generated overwhelming feedback. Here is more information of the same focus.

In the South Pacific Island of Fiji, "Fat Phobia" has begun to plague its inhabitants, ever since satellite T.V. beamed its way into their lives. In the traditional Fijian culture, food is typically rich with coconut cream and the ideal body is large and robust. The Fijians refer to weight loss as "going thin," and is cause for alarm and concern for one's health. In a survey of 65 Fijian girls averaging 17 years old, Dr. Anne Becker, research director at the Harvard Eating Disorder Center, found that those who watched T.V. three or more nights per week were 50% more likely to feel "too big and fat."

In the six years since television has made its appearance, not only are the South Sea teens adopting the clothing and hairstyles of Western women, but they are unfortunately showing serious signs of eating disorders as well. 15% of the Fijian teens surveyed said they had vomited to control their weight, compared to just 3% in 1995, when T.V. first arrived. The teens cited shows such as "Melrose Place" and "Beverly Hills 90210" as inspiration for wanting to change their bodies.

Based on these facts, one doesn't need a research degree to figure out the possible effects of a lifetime of television watching! Take this challenge—turn off the T.V. and tune into yourself. There you will find the truth.

WOMEN'S ISSUES

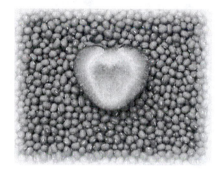

PMS

MOST WOMEN, SOMETIME IN THEIR LIVES, will have a problem with Premenstrual Syndrome—a condition with a wide variety of complaints that generally surfaces from 2 to 10 days prior to menstruation. Research has shown that diet and nutritional status are related to PMS. Women who drink caffeine or alcohol, eat refined sugar, salt and excess animal fats may be creating more severe symptoms. Adequate protein (1 gram per 2 pounds of body weight) helps the adrenal glands manage stress, and fresh fruits, leafy green vegetables, legumes, seeds, whole grains and cereal supply the necessary vitamins, minerals and carbohydrates.

Exercise plays an important role in the reduction of symptoms. Twenty to thirty minutes of uninterrupted exercise per day helps balance the hormones—estrogen and progesterone. It improves circulation and is a good release for frustration, anxiety and depression.

Evening primrose oil and Vitamin B-6 have been reported to improve conditions of PMS, as do the herbs Dong Quai and Black Cohosh. Magnesium also plays an interesting role. In PMS sufferers with low blood sugar, magnesium can decrease the response of insulin so that those dreaded monthly sugar cravings aren't as difficult to manage. Magnesium helps to relax the muscles and may diminish cramping.

Avoid high-sodium foods. Diuretics are not the answer. Initially they may ease water retention, but if taken for a long time or in high dosages they can have dangerous side effects, including dizziness, nausea, electrolyte imbalanced, even lung and kidney failure.

By using exercise, proper diet, and sensible supplementation, many women may alleviate their monthly bout with PMS.

MENOPAUSE IS
A NATURAL PROCESS

MY MOM LOVED SAYING "I'm not having a hot flash, I'm having a power surge." Recently, I saw a bumper sticker that said "I'm out of estrogen and I have a gun!" Menopause, also referred to as "the change," is indeed an interesting time of life.

As women approach age 48–52 (although some women begin earlier or stop later), basically the ovaries age, shrink and ovulation stops, resulting in an end to menstruation. This is menopause. Simply put, menopause is a hormone deficiency condition. When the hormones estrogen, progesterone and androgens begin to decline during peri-menopause (the 7 to 10 years leading up to menopause), a host of symptoms occur. The major concerns include: hot flashes, insomnia, joint/muscle ache, weight gain, fatigue, loss of muscle and skin tone and mental confusion. The hormone balance that once assisted with soft skin, normal mood and a healthy sex drive becomes skewed. Some symptoms naturally fade away in time, while others remain. There are a number of tried and true nutritional recommendations and lifestyle changes that, not only ease the discomfort of menopause, but support the entire body to ensure years of good health.

The Right Diet

The goal is to eat an easily digested, lowfat, high fiber, nutrient rich diet. Plant based foods can actually mimic the action of estrogen, thus creating fewer menopausal symptoms. Eat lots of the following for beneficial hormonal balance:

- Fresh organic fruits and vegetables (the more the merrier)
- Whole grains, such as RyVita crackers or Ezekiel bread
- Raw nuts (small amounts)
- Range-fed poultry
- Cold water fish, such as salmon and tuna
- Flaxseed oil (1–2 Tbsp/day) or ground flaxseed (2–5 Tbsp/day)
- Raw seeds (pumpkin, sesame, sunflower can also be made into nut butters)
- Beans (put kidney beans and garbanzos on your salad)
- Water! (8 glasses per day, helps with everything!)
- Green foods (such as spirulina, chlorella, barley greens and blue-green algae 1–2 Tbsp/day mixed in water, fruit shakes or smoothies)
- Tofu (non GMO) 50–150mg/day. Scientific research continues to indicate that soy based products help protect women in mid-life. If allergic to soy, take soy isoflavones in capsule form (50–60mg/day)

The Wrong Diet

- Too many dairy products: The main dietary source of arachidonic acid, a type of fat that can result in fluid retention, bloating and cramps.
- Sugar: One of the hardest things to give up, but one of the most beneficial. Sweets act as an irritant to the body, cause toxins to accumulate and make the body work harder. A high insulin level has also been related to increased release of xenoestrogens linked to female cancers.
- Alcohol: The chemical ETOH, ethyl alcohol, causes increased fat stores in the liver decreasing our blood's purification system.
- Red meat: Menopausal women often store fat, rather than burn it for energy, because their metabolism slows. Red meat is high in saturated fat. This leads to obesity and heart disease.
- Wheat products: Gluten, which is the protein found in wheat, is highly allergenic and difficult for the body to break down. During menopause, digestion slows and wheat products can cause greater intolerance on one's system.

More Menopausal Suggestions

- Physical Activity: Exercise helps with every menopausal symptom and slows down the aging process. Moderate aerobic exercise such as walking, swimming or biking (30 minutes, 5 times a week), as well as lifting weights, or doing yoga (1–2 times a week) can help build lost muscle and keep bones strong. Even gardening can count as physical activity.
- Supplementation: According to Susan Lark, MD, a leading specialist on women's health, to calm and balance estrogen activity take:
  - Quercerin (100–600mg/day)
  - Vitamin C (1000–3000mg/day)
  - Vitamin E (d-alpha tocopherol 400–2000IU/day)
  - Vitamin A (Beta Carotene 5000–12000IU/day)
- Hot flash relief: Black cohosh (standardized extract 40–60mg/day)
- Heavy period and erratic cycles during peri-menopause. Chaste Tree Berry or Vitex (175mg extract)
- Insomnia Relief: Kava root (140mg before bed)

INSULIN AND BREAST CANCER

I AM WRITING THIS IN HONOR OF MY MOTHER who died on Memorial Day 1999 of breast cancer. She had a double mastectomy in 1978 and was disease-free for 21 years until a reoccurrence claimed her life.

In what appears to be a strong, new risk factor for progression of breast cancer, a recent Canadian study involving 535 women followed over a ten-year period, demonstrated that high levels of insulin in the blood is an ominous sign for women with the disease. Women with breast cancer and high levels of insulin were about eight times more likely to develop recurrence and die of the disease as women who had normal insulin levels.

A hormone developed in the pancreas, insulin, is critical in controlling the blood sugar level needed for energy. Simple carbohydrates we consume, typically in the form of white flour, sugar and refined starches, create excess glucose in the system which not only stresses the body, but over time can result in the cells becoming less responsive to insulin. This condition, known as insulin resistance, is estimated to affect half of the American population! Aside from the recent breast cancer findings, it's wise to keep the blood sugar level balanced for a number of other health reasons.

Some keys to maintaining a stable insulin level include:

- Eat foods that have a lower glycemic index which lowers insulin producing potential. Since 1986, the food plan advocated by **The Healthy Way** has done just this!

- Eating throughout the day helps prevent the "starvation response," which results in more insulin being produced. At The Healthy Way we offer a chewable supplement made of chromium and B vitamins that helps maintain insulin levels.

- Exercise helps to keep insulin levels more stable. Find a personal fitness trainer and/or a group class to help get you moving.

- Stay away from, or greatly limit your intake of sugar and artificial sweeteners. There are good tasting, healthier options, like Stevia, to satisfy the sweet tooth.

- Eat "colorful" foods. White foods, such as white potatoes, white rice, white flour and all foods made from them are less nutritious and more insulin producing that their "colored" counterparts.

- Remember to eat breakfast. The name literally means "to break the fast." Insulin levels typically don't peak and valley as much when breakfast is consumed. Get into the breakfast habit if you aren't already doing so.

We have lost far too many of our mothers, sisters and friends to the dreaded disease of breast cancer. Mammography is helpful for early detection, but no conclusive research has offered an effective prevention program. Until the cause of breast cancer is found, I think it wise to adopt as many health promoting strategies as possible.

MOTHERLY ADVICE

W E HAVE LOST FAR TOO MANY of our mothers and sisters to breast cancer. The following is another suggested protection plan, all unproven as of yet, but nevertheless benign in its implementation and what I personally practice.

Protection Plan

1. **Avoid petroleum products and pesticides,** both of which are suspected to be "endocrine disrupters," (also known as xenoestrogens) known to interfere with the action of hormones in the body. Scientists have consistently found that an elevated estrogen level can promote cancerous breast tumors.

2. **Avoid hydrogenated or partially hydrogenated oils** (also know as transfats) in your diet, as they act as magnets for free radicals. Researchers have actually found these man-made fats in the tissue of malignant breast tumors. Read the labels on packaged foods and make the wisest choices.

3. **Microwave in glass or ceramic only.** When plastic is heated, it can migrate into the food and thus create a potent carcinogen.

4. **Do not use anti-perspirants.** Use deodorant instead. The majority of breast tumors are in the upper, outer quadrant of the breast...near the armpit. Antiperspirants inhibit the normal lymphatic drainage of toxins via underarm sweat. Why wait 5 or 10 years for researchers to discover this as a potential cause? Switch to plain deodorant and underarm shield guards if necessary.

5. **Go braless once in a while.** Two sociological studies have theorized that the possible reason African and Japanese women have such low incidence of breast cancer is because they do not routinely wear bras, especially underwire bras that may constrict the lymphatic drainage of the mammary glands. Again, this is pure speculation, but an easy and possibly relaxing suggestion that can cause no harm.

6. **Take Calcium D-glucarate.** This mineral has been shown to metabolize excess estrogen in the body. It's available at **The Healthy Way** and most supplement stores.

7. **Eat at least four servings of any of the following crucifer vegetables every week:** broccoli, cauliflower, asparagus, cabbage or brussel sprouts. If you don't like vegetables, then make a "green drink" using such products as "pro greens" or "green magma." This way you won't miss your daily greens.

8. **Stay lean.** Fat cells produce estrogen and also suppress the immune system. A body composition of 25% body fat or lower is best for most women.

9. **Nurse your babies.** Women who have never nursed, have an increased risk of breast cancer.

10. **Avoid smoking, and avoid or limit alcohol intake.**

Another substance worth mentioning is di-indole methane (DIM). If either your mother or a sister have a history of breast cancer, there may be a genetically abnormal imbalance of estrogen metabolites, called the 2/16 alpha-hydroxy-estrone ratio. DIM is the active ingredient of cruciferous vegetables that has been shown to modulate and correct this imbalance.

MORE MOTHERLY ADVICE

IN WRITING A PIECE ABOUT BREAST CANCER PROTECTION, I received overwhelming feedback. It was obvious from the calls and comments that many of you believe, until medicine finds "the cure," why not implement unproven, yet harmless steps to reduce the risk of breast cancer? Here are a few more suggestions in reducing risk factors.

Recommendations

1. **Eat soy products.** Researchers estimate approximately 60% of cancer in US women is attributed to dietary factors. By incorporating soy into the diet, potent cancer fighting compounds such as protease inhibitors can turn off the signals that tell malignant cells to multiply. Beneficial soy products include:

   ¾ cup of soybeans, 4–5 ounces of tofu, 8–10 ounces of soymilk and/or supplements that contains isoflavones (50mg/day). Be sure to purchase "GMO-free" soy products.

2. **Say yes to broccoli.** Cruciferous vegetables, especially broccoli, contain numerous anti-cancer properties, as well as hormone regulating factors. Eat it at least 2–3 times per week.

3. **Flaxseed or fish oil.** Studies have shown that women with high levels of the Omega-3 essential fatty acids have a lower risk of breast cancer. Two to three tablespoons of freshly ground flaxseed (in a coffee grinder) sprinkled on salads, cereal, juice or water does the trick. Salad dressing can be made with flaxseed oil or one can take a fish oil capsule (1000 to 2000mg/day is the suggested preventative dosage).

4. **Use caution with dry cleaning.** Commercial dry cleaning methods employ a highly toxic, carcinogenic chemical called perchloroethylene (Perc), that is known to be a hormone disrupter. Look for a "green" cleaner, one that uses water and steam based methods. At the very least, tell your cleaners not to wrap your clothes in plastic, or if they are plastic wrapped, let your clothing air out before bringing them into your closet.

5. **Exercise!** Research shows again and again that 30 minutes per day of exercise is not just good for the heart, but breasts as well! People who exercise (brisk walk is fine) have a lower incidence of cancer.

6. **More fiber please.** Make plant foods the center of your diet. Eat a variety of organic fruits and vegetables. By doing so, it speeds the transit through the bowel, limiting the exposure time to carcinogens, as well as reducing the amount of circulating estrogen, which decreases the risk of breast cancer.

BREAST CANCER PROTECTION PLAN

I AM SURE MOST OF YOU ARE WELL AWARE of the threat that breast cancer poses to all women. The San Francisco Bay Area unfortunately possesses one of the highest breast cancer rates in the U.S. The news isn't all bad though. Statistics can be misleading. The current statistic that 1 out of 8 women will succumb to breast cancer is based on living to the age of 85. My mom, who was struck with bilateral breast cancer remained disease-free for 22 years.

As with all cancer, there is much more to be learned. Fortunately, some of the risk factors associated with breast cancer have been well defined, many of which are within our control. We know, for example, that the incidence of breast cancer in Japanese women eating the traditional diet (high in soy products) is one quarter that of U.S. women. Two phytocompounds, found in soy, which offer protective mechanisms are isoflavones and genistein.

Research has consistently shown that an elevated estrogen level can promote malignant breast tumors.

Your Breast Cancer Protective Plan

1. Petroleum-based products are potent carcinogens. Do not use pesticides, herbicides or fungicides in your garden. Avoid bug sprays and flea bombs. Most petroleum-based products used today are estrogen analogs (xenoestrogens) which have been highly suspected to cause breast cancer.

2. Buy organic produce because washing with water doesn't remove pesticides.

3. Decrease dietary fats, sugars and processed foods. Decrease or omit alcohol. Eat soy products 2–3 times per week. All the above can affect the estrogen level.

4. Exercise can decrease estrogen levels. Women who work out consistently have a lower risk factor.

5. High fiber diet—eat whole grains, fresh fruits and vegetables. Add 1½ cups of oat bran or 1 tsp. psyllium to yogurt, juice or water for extra protection.

6. Lose weight. Fatty tissue produces estrogen, even after menopause.

Still in question…X-rays, synthetic hormone replacement therapy and electromagnetic fields. They say knowledge is power, so let's learn all we can to implement a breast cancer prevention plan.

EXERCISE

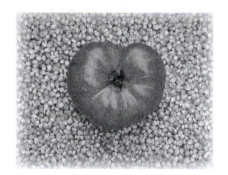

THE BENEFITS OF
EXERCISING ARE ENDLESS

WITHOUT QUESTION, EXERCISE IS ESSENTIAL TO HEALTH. It helps everything from sleep to looking and feeling better. By combining a low calorie, nutritious diet with a regular exercise program, you'll be more successful than trying either step alone. The benefits of exercise actually go far beyond that of calories burned as a result of increased physical activity. It can also:

- Strengthen the immune system
- Increase energy level
- Decrease total body fat.
- Reduce cholesterol levels and triglyceride levels in the blood.
- Lower blood sugar level.
- Increase muscle strength and endurance.
- Improve the efficiency of the lungs, heart, and circulatory system.
- Strengthen tendons and ligaments.
- Improve one's attitude and self esteem.

Try a variety of different exercises geared to benefit all parts of the body. Find something you enjoy doing. I do weight resistance exercise and enjoy using my home treadmill, but swimming is my real joy. Try exercising to music or working out with a friend to spark interest and alleviate boredom. Most important, *Start Today!!!*

"Desserts" Spelled Backward Is "Stressed"

J UST HOW MUCH EXERCISE does it take to work off a 300 calorie indulgence? Probably a lot more time than it took to consume those calories. The following chart may give you some idea of the work required to justify that extra piece of cake or pie you couldn't resist at your last meal.

⅛ chocolate cream pie (300 calories) = 60 minutes of brisk walking.

½₂ devil's food cake (189 calories) = 50 minutes of gardening.

⅛ homemade pumpkin pie (241 calories) = 40 minutes of chopping wood.

1 square homemade brownie w/nuts, no frosting (97 calories) = 20 minutes of rowing.

1 square gingerbread from mix (174 Calories) = 44 minutes of bicycling (5.5 mph).

⅛ lite cheesecake (210 calories) = 30 minutes of tennis.

1 granola bar (109 calories) = 11 minutes of swimming.

1 piece homemade angel food cake, no frosting (161 calories) = 24 minutes of digging with a hand shovel.

A little trivia: *"Reach for your mate instead of a plate"*

Kissing can burn up about 12 calories

15 minutes of love-making typically burns 63 calories.

THE WONDERS OF WALKING

EXERCISE RESEARCHERS HAVE CONCLUDED that walking may be the perfect exercise. Not running or aerobics or trips to the gym, but good old simple, inexpensive, readily available walking. A study recently conducted at the University of Colorado in Boulder compared walking, running and step aerobics and found similar fitness gains when all exercisers worked at the same intensity level. The only difference? Runners lost an average of eleven workout days due to injury; walkers lost only one and a half. What gets most people motivated to start a walking program is the hope of thinner thighs or a slimmer midsection. Over the last decade, dozens of studies have shown that regular walking offers enormous health benefits, as well as the physical improvement.

It increases lung power, strengthens the heart, improves circulation, strengthens bones, reduces blood pressure, relieves stress, decreases body fat and appetite, reduces the risk of diabetes, colon cancer and gallstones. The list goes on and on. Walking has also been shown to be an effective mood enhancer and is one of the few exercises that doesn't inhibit conversation. Dr. Joann Manson, Chief of Preventive Medicine at Harvard's Brigham and Women's Hospital stated, "If everyone in the U.S. were to walk briskly 30 minutes a day, we could cut the incidence of many chronic diseases 30% to 40%."

The goal is to walk at a reasonably vigorous clip, a pace as if you're late for dinner at your in-law's house. Aim for a 12 minute mile (4–5 m.p.h) for 30 minutes 5 or 6 times a week. For an extra intensity boost, walk hills or use walking poles which increase the calorie expenditure by an average of 25%. Poles are also useful if one needs to decrease stress upon the legs and feet. To get the upper body into the act, bend the arms at about a 90º degree angle so they'll swing faster and keep elbows close to the midsection. Walking with hand weights can throw off stride and strain muscles. Wrist weights, no more than 3 pounds, seem to work better. Wearing ankle weights frequently causes injury to the knees, hips and lower back.

Pay attention to your shoes, which need more room at the front for feet to spread. Drink water to stay hydrated, ideally ½ glass (4 oz) every 15 minutes. Three to four big swigs from a sipper or water bottle would achieve this. Remember to start out a walking program slowly, incorporating warm-up and cool down stretches. Walking with a friend or at a specific time each day may work best. Other folks plug in walking whenever they can, such as parking a few blocks away from the store and walking back with the bags, or taking the stairs rather than the elevator.

Walking won't cure everything that ails you, but it probably is as close to a magic bullet as we will come in modern medicine.

Exercise ❤

HOLIDAYS vs. HOLI-DAZE

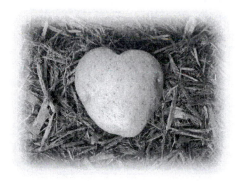

THE HUNGRY GHOST

HALLOWEEN IS A CELEBRATION marked by candy, sweets and tasty treats. It also signifies the grand opening of the annual "free style eating season," where most of us will innocently continue to gain weight until January 1.

Growing up as a "pleasingly plump" little girl, Halloween was a big event for me. My candy bag never lasted as long as everyone else's. I could never get my fill of treats! As the years have passed, my sweet tooth has subsided...thanks, primarily to greater awareness of how sugar negatively affects me, learning how to control my insulin/blood sugar level, exercise, therapy and limiting the amount of sugar in my diet.

Nevertheless, when October 31 rolls around, that hungry ghost inside (and in most weight-challenged folk) still comes out to haunt me a bit! After years of "testing", I now fully realize when I eat candy I will gain weight. Period! It took so very long to finally come to this simple truth. I'd use every excuse in the book..."I haven't eaten all day so this won't matter;" "Ohhh just this little bit couldn't possibly hurt;""Heck, it's only Halloween one time a year."

The fact remains, when I eat candy or sweets, the scale goes up. If I'm willing to do the extra work it takes to get the candy weight off, then I'll eat some. If not, then I remember it was sugar and excuses that caused me to be chubby in the first place and it still holds true today.

If you are eating more of your kid's Halloween candy than they are, or if the leftover candy you passed out is still around and calling your name...it may signal a need for help. By breaking the cycle of blood sugar fluctuation you can effectively deal with putting the hungry ghost to rest...once and for all!

HERE COME THE PARTIES

HISTORY TELLS US THAT MOST AMERICANS GAIN WEIGHT over the holidays. With the abundance of treats, endless social functions and added stressors (family dramas, extended travel and financial concerns), it's little wonder our waistlines expand. Here are a few strategies to navigate through those festive times without suffering the consequences.

- Make sure you have a well-balanced snack before you leave for the event. A protein shake or energy bar with at least 15 gms. protein, no more than 20 gms. fat, and less than 10 gms. carbo would help to provide insurance.

- Stand away from the buffet table and be selective about the foods you choose.

- Remember that you and only you are in control of your life. Make a commitment before going to the party. Each time you successfully deal with a different eating situation, you gain more willpower, feel more confident and become more self-assured. Think of the satisfaction of actually losing or maintaining your weight between Thanksgiving and New Year's.

- People seldom notice what you're eating or not eating if you don't draw attention to the fact that you are dieting.

- Most holiday entertainers offer a selection of foods for weight conscious individuals. If nothing is served that is compatible with your food plan, just take a small portion. Keep in mind that the purpose of getting together with family and friends is to enjoy one another's company and have a good time. Eating doesn't have to be the main event. Let the good conversation fill you.

- If the foods in the meal are rich and full of sugars or creams, take a small portion and leave some on your plate. Fill up on the salad, fruit, and vegetables.

- Most foods are tasted for only three seconds, then they are either used to replenish the body or stored as fat. The first bite tastes the same as the last bite!

- Use a smaller plate. Not only does it aid with portion control, but you can fool your brain (and stomach) into feeling satisfied with less food.

- Candlelight isn't the smartest weight loss technique. Researchers at UC Irvine found more binge activity and unconscious eating took place in low-light environments. So, if you are at a party, stay in the well-lit areas.

HAPPY THANKSGIVING

EVERY HUMAN NEEDS TO CELEBRATE, and in most cultures food plays a part in the festivities. Thanksgiving was never meant to be a day of going without, of calculating calories, and fussing over bad fats versus good fats. Nor was it ever intended to be a day of gluttonous mass consumption, where you feel as gassy and full as a balloon in the Macy's Thanksgiving Day Parade! **Moderation,** the art of staying somewhere in the middle, is the key. Sure your calorie intake may be higher, but one day of overeating has never made anyone fat. Here are a few strategies for staying in balance on the big day:

- Bring an entrée or hors d'oeuvres that you can freely indulge in. Prepare a fresh vegetable tray served with a lowfat or nonfat dip that you can munch on all day. Make deviled eggs using prepared mustard and lowfat/no-sugar mayonnaise. Boil up some jumbo prawns and serve with cocktail sauce, lemon, and horseradish or salsa.

- If turkey is being served, eat the white meat only, which has 10 gms. less fat and a 100 calories less than the same amount of dark meat. It is okay to leave the skin on while cooking poultry to maintain moisture. However, once cooked, avoid eating the skin and dark meat.

- Do not starve all day in preparation for your Thanksgiving feast. Study after study clearly shows that when one goes without food, the blood sugar (insulin level) drops, thus creating more cravings and a slower metabolic rate.

- Do not eat a food just because it is on your plate. Eat slowly and set down your utensils frequently. Try to make a meal last for twenty minutes, as that is the length of time it takes before the hunger center in the brain can register fullness. Cut your food in small pieces and chew it thoroughly.

- When drinking alcohol, try to make each cocktail last an hour. For the weight concerned, wine is the alcoholic beverage of choice because it has the least amount of calories (70 cals. for white and 74 cals. for red). Alternating between cocktails with a glass of water is a good habit to follow.
- Be careful when preparing foods. Don't taste test your way into extra pounds. Remember those little tastes add up. Chew gum or have some raw veggies to decrease unconscious eating.
- Do not salt foods. Salt is an acquired taste. The more salt you eat, the more you want! Be aware that an additional ¼ teaspoon of salt equals ½ pound of water being retained by the body.
- Exercise early in the day. New findings show that the metabolic benefits continue long after you have completed your exercise.
- If the choice is mashed potatoes or sweet potatoes, go for the tuber. One cup mashed potatoes with one tablespoon butter is more fat and calories than the sweet potatoes, even if topped with brown sugar and marshmallows.
- Have the piece of pecan pie (450 calories) if that's what you really want. Just remember to forego the unconsciously devoured handfuls of mixed nuts (407 calories for ½ cup) on the hors d'ouevres table earlier in the day.

GUILT~FREE RECIPES

For Americans, Thanksgiving is considered the biggest food event of the year. According to the Calorie Control Council, a traditional holiday dinner, with all the trimmings, adds up to more than 4500 calories and 229 grams of fat! You can enjoy a holiday feast without packing on the pounds.

Here are a few traditional holiday recipes, pared down to be "*Healthy Way Style*" and guaranteed to please the most discriminating of taste buds!

Mushroom Caps *(makes 1–2 servings)*

½ lb. mushrooms (approximately 12–15 medium size mushrooms)
4 Ryvita crackers
1 (3½ oz.) can crab meat
1 green onion, minced
garlic powder
salt and pepper, to taste
Remove stems from mushrooms and microwave for 2 to 3 minutes to soften. Place the Ryvita crackers, mushroom stems, garlic powder, crab meat, green onion, salt, and pepper into a blender or food processor and mix. Fill the mushroom caps with the mixture and bake for 8–10 minutes at 350°.

Red Pepper Dip *(makes 2 cups)*

4 red bell peppers, quartered
8 oz. plain nonfat yogurt or fat-free sour cream
1 pkg. vegetable soup mix (such as Spice Hunter or Knorr)
Blend all ingredients together in a food processor. This red dip looks especially nice served in a red or green cabbage, hollowed-out and cut flat along the bottom to act as a serving bowl.

Cranberry Jello Mold *(makes 6–8 servings)*

1 medium orange, ground up with skin
¾ cup port wine
1 (3 oz.) pkg. sugar-free raspberry Jello
1 (8 oz. can whole cranberries
¼ cup walnuts, chopped (optional)
Boil port wine and ground orange together for 1–2 minutes. Pour hot mixture into bowl with Jello, cranberries, and nuts. Pour into gelatin mold. Chill. Serve when firm.

Sweet Potato Pumpkins *(makes 8 servings)*

    1 lb. baked sweet potatoes, peeled & quarter cut

    8 oz. drained, canned, crushed pineapple

    1 egg

    ½ cup cranberry sauce (natural fruit sweetened)

    2 tsp. "Butter Buds" (or equivalent)

    ¼ tsp. ground nutmeg

    ¼ tsp. pepper

    8 mini pumpkins (hollowed out)

Whip together the potatoes, pineapple, egg, spices and seasonings. Swirl in the cranberry sauce. Bake the mixture @ 375° for 20 minutes. Then transfer potato mixture into the center of each mini pumpkin and place into a 9 x 13 dish with about ½ – 1 inch of water. Bake at 375° for an additional 10–15 minutes. Garnish with parsley. The pumpkin top and stem can be used for a fancy presentation.

Healthy Gravy Makings

The key to making low-fat gravies is to decrease the turkey drippings. Place the drippings in a large zip-lock heavy-duty plastic bag. Begin draining the drippings into a 4-cup measure or large bowl. Cover and refrigerate the drippings until ready to use them.

Smooth & Creamy Turkey Gravy *(makes 2 ⅓ cups)*

    1 T. peanut oil

    3 T. all-purpose whole wheat flour

    1 cup low sodium fat free chicken broth

    1 cup degreased turkey drippings

    ¼ cup Chablis or other dry white wine

    ¼ tsp. salt

Heat oil in a medium size heavy saucepan over medium heat. Stir in flour, cook one minute, stirring constantly with a wire whisk. Gradually add other ingredients, stirring constantly. Bring to a boil. Reduce heat, and simmer, uncovered for 2 minutes or until mixture is slightly thickened.

Sage Dressing *(makes 2 servings)*

2 T. oat bran
4 Wasa or Ryvita crackers
2 T. onion, chopped
1 stalk celery, sliced
1 apple, shredded with peel
2–3 tsp. sage
¼ tsp. each poultry seasoning and celery flakes
1 egg white
dash Butter Buds
dash pepper
1 T. onion flakes
vegetable oil spray

In a food processor, grind oat bran and crackers. In a lightly oiled pan, sauté onion and celery until tender. Cool. Combine all ingredients in a bowl and mix well. Place into a small, sprayed baking dish and bake at 375° for 35 minutes.

Spinach Barley Stuffing *(makes 4 cups)*

1 cup onion, minced
1 cup fresh mushrooms, sliced
3 cups cooked barley
2 Ryvita crackers, ground
2 cloves garlic, minced
1 tsp. dried whole basil
¼ tsp. dried summer savory
¼ tsp. paprika
¼ tsp. ground nutmeg
¼ tsp. pepper
2 egg whites, slightly beaten
1 (10 oz.) package frozen chopped spinach, thawed and drained
1 T. peanut oil

Heat oil in a large nonstick skillet over medium high heat. Add onion and mushrooms. Sauté until tender. Remove from heat. Add remaining ingredients and stir well. Place mixture inside turkey breast or in a lightly oiled baking dish. Bake at 375° for 20–30 minutes.

Holiday Pumpkin Pie *(makes 4 servings)*

Pie Crust

8 Ryvita crackers
1 green apple, grated with peel
1 egg, beaten
dash each cinnamon and nutmeg
1 tsp. sweetener (optional)
1 tsp. butter extract
vegetable spray

Finely grind crackers in food processor. Add remaining ingredients. Pat into a 9-inch sprayed pie pan. Bake at 350° for 15 minutes. Set aside to cool while filling is prepared.

Filling

2 pkg. unflavored gelatin

4 T. nonfat dry milk

1 ½ cups water

2 eggs, beaten

1 (16 oz.) can pumpkin puree

¼ cup protein powder

2–3 T. sweetener

2 T. pumpkin pie spice

½ tsp. each cinnamon, ginger, and maple flavoring

Place gelatin and powdered milk in water and dissolve over low heat in a saucepan. Set aside to cool. In a large bowl, mix eggs, pumpkin, protein powder, sweetener, spices, and gelatin mixture. Pour into a baking dish and bake at 350° for 35 minutes. When cool, but not set hard, put into baked pie shell and chill. Top with whipped topping.

Tofu Pumpkin Pudding (makes 8 servings)

1 box Fearn bran muffin mix

⅓ cup applesauce

1 egg

1 ½ boxes Mori-Nu extra-firm lite tofu

1 (15 oz) can pumpkin puree

½ tsp. stevia powder

1 tsp. vanilla

1 T. pumpkin pie spice or next 4 ingredients:

 1 ½ tsp. ground cinnamon

 ¾ tsp. ground ginger

 ¼ tsp. ground nutmeg

 ¼ tsp. ground cloves

Crust

Mix Fearn bran muffin mix, applesauce, and 1 egg. Press into 8-inch pie pan. Bake 5 minutes in a 425 degree oven. Cool crust.

Filling

Blend tofu in food processor or blender until smooth. Add remaining ingredients and blend well. Pour into pie shell. Bake for approximately 1 hour. Filling will be soft, but will set as it chills. Chill and serve.

The specialty items that appear in these recipes are available at **The Healthy Way** or your local healthfood store. We also have a wonderful cookbook, *Cooking the Healthy Way*, filled with taste treats that are easy to prepare and fit the bill as genuine health food.

Happy Thanksgiving to Everyone!

Holidays ♥

BAKING FOR THE HOLIDAYS

Thoughts of the holiday season conjure up images of fireside gatherings, sweet smells of cinnamon, peppermint and nostalgic times with family and friends. But it also brings thoughts of panic if you are trying to stay in control and keep your weight down. These guidelines may help:

- If you typically make dozens of holiday cookies, bake them ahead of time and store them in the freezer or in sealed containers. Why not bake fewer cookies this year or forget the whole tradition altogether, especially if tempted by freshly baked treats. Other homemade items that can be packaged festively and that are well received include: pickled red bell peppers, all fruit jam, spaghetti sauce, homemade soap, herbed vinegars...the list goes on. It doesn't have to be a fattening gift.

- Try baking only enough for each occasion by making the dough ahead of time, forming it into rolls and refrigerating it. Before company comes, simply cut off what you need and bake only enough for that occasion. The dough will keep for weeks in the refrigerator and your company will get fresh baked cookies. More importantly, you won't have cookies around to tempt you.

- Modify your favorite recipes to cut calories from fat and sugar without sacrificing taste and texture. This is easy and works well for most recipes. However, it may take some experimentation to see just how much fat and sugar can be reduced before there is a noticeable change in texture or flavor. Fat (butter, oil or shortening) in recipes can generally be cut a ¼ to ½ before noticing the difference in a baked product. In recipes calling for 1 cup butter or oil, for instance, 1 cup of unsweetened applesauce can be substituted. Sugar may be cut ⅓ to ½ before there is a change in sweetness or texture. Unconstituted organic, frozen apple juice concentrate may be used in lieu of sugar as a healthier substitute in recipes.

By making a few changes in recipes and reorganizing previous ways of doing things to better support health and weight loss goals, you can still enjoy holiday treats. It's all about choice. You can pass up the sweets, you can eat them or you can choose one of the many low calorie alternatives that are just as satisfying.

TAKE THIS TEST

THE TYPICAL AMERICAN puts on an average of four to seven pounds between Thanksgiving and New Year's Day. Did you gain weight over the holiday season?

Yes   No

At the turn of the century, approximately 3 lbs. of sugar per year were consumed by the average American. Now, 100 years later, the typical sugar intake exceeds 125 lbs. per person per year. Did you overdo it with sweets & fats in the past few months (or perhaps the past few years??)

Yes   No

When sugars & simple carbohydrates are eaten in excess, oftentimes one experiences a decreased immunity, depression & strong cravings for more sweets. Do you have, or have you recently had, a cold? Perhaps you can't seem to shake a bug?

Yes   No

With the holidays behind us, have you had a difficult time eliminating sweets from your diet? Do you have the Post-Holiday Blues?

Yes   No

HAPPY NEW YOU!

OK! NOW THAT THE LAST OF THE CHEESEBALLS, RUMBALLS AND EGGNOG have been "over indulged upon..."it is time to get back to the business of eating for health. **The Healthy Way's** Cleansing Diet is a tried and true food plan, designed to detoxify and cleanse the system. By following the regimen anywhere from 3 to 7 days, the bloat, lethargy and extra pounds picked up over the holidays will quickly subside.

Cleansing Diet

Upon rising: 8 oz. warm water w/ 2 Tbsp. lemon juice

Within one hour of rising: Select 1 protein serving from the following:

- 2 eggs
- ½ cup nonfat/sugar free cottage cheese
- 1 cup plain, nonfat yogurt
- 1 RyVita cracker

8 oz. water or herbal tea

Mid morning: Select 1 fruit serving from the following:

- 1 medium apple, orange or grapefruit
- 1 cup berries
- 1 cup melon

8 oz. water

Lunch: Select 1 protein serving of:

- 3–5 oz. poultry, fish, or lean beef
- 1–2 cups steamed veggies
- Green beans, broccoli, zucchini, asparagus, spinach or cauliflower
- Large green salad
- 2 Tbsp. oil and vinegar and lemon juice to taste

8 oz. water

Mid-afternoon:

- ½ cup nonfat/sugar free cottage cheese or 1 to 2 part-skim string cheese
- 1 Ryvita cracker

8 oz. water

Dinner:	Select 1 protein serving from the following:

- 3–5 oz. poultry, fish, or lean beef
- 1–2 cups steamed veggies
- Green beans, broccoli, zucchini, asparagus, spinach or cauliflower
- ½ cups cooked brown rice or 1 yam/sweet potato

8 oz. water

After Dinner: Select 1 fruit serving from the following:

- 1 medium apple, orange or grapefruit
- 1 cup berries
- 1 cup melon

8 oz. water

At bedtime: 8 oz. water or herbal tea

Helpful Hints

- Eat food in the order listed.
- Stop if you are full.
- Drink 64 oz. of water daily.
- No juice. Eat the fruit for fiber.
- If hungry eat 1 hard boiled egg or 1 oz. string cheese up to 3 times a day.
- Do not eat two to three hours before bedtime.
- One cup of coffee daily, preferably decaf, if necessary.

For Vegetarians

Protein can be:

- 5 ounces of lite 1% tofu
- 2 scoops of low carb, no sugar protein powder
- ½ cup cottage cheese (nonfat/lowfat)
- 1 cup plain, nonfat yogurt

MOTIVATION

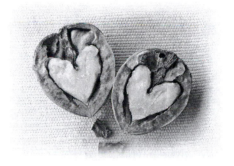

MOTIVATORS

GOOD NEWS IS ALWAYS LIKE A BREATH OF FRESH AIR. Here is an offering of positive sentiments I've collected over the years, a few even from fortune cookies!

- Do not wish to be anything but who you are and try to be that perfectly.
- Why not go out on a limb...isn't that where all the fruit is?
- Attitudes are contagious..is yours worth catching?
- The race is not always to the swift, but to those who keep on running.
- Some people dream of worthy accomplishments, while others stay awake and do them.
- You cannot discover new oceans unless you have the courage to lose sight of the shore.
- Keep a green tree in your heart and the songbird will come.
- Energy and persistence will conquer all things.
- See opportunity in every difficulty.
- If you're not riding the wave of change, you'll find yourself beneath it.
- Accept the challenges so that you may feel the exhilaration of victory.
- All you need to give to be a winner, is all you have.
- We are what we repeatedly do. Excellence is not an act, but a habit.
- Think you can, think you can't; either way, you'll be right.
- Kindness gives birth to kindness.
- Knock the "t" off the "can't"
- Enthusiasm *IS* life.
- Hope is putting faith to work when doubting would be easier.
- To dream of the person you would like to be, is to waste the person you are.

RESOLUTION POWER

SOME OF THE STEPS TO SEE A GOAL BECOME REALITY ARE SIMPLE, yet powerful tools. Here are suggestions that will improve the likelihood of success.

1. Tell someone about the goal. Nothing will help you achieve your goals like accountability. When you tell your spouse and /or friend about your goals, you will have to answer at some point, the inevitable question of whether or not you reached your objective. This is a powerful motivating factor.

2. Set your daily priorities according to your goals. When you prioritize the tasks you must do each day, ask yourself one question: How will doing this task (or not doing it) affect my being able to reach the goals I've set for myself? Those tasks that have a direct impact should be moved up to the top of the priority list, while those that have little impact on reaching your goals can be moved down the list.

3. Visualize the achievement of your goal. If your goal is to lose weight, find a picture of a slender person and put it where you will see it several times throughout the day. To make it even more realistic, many people will actually take the head of a photograph of themselves and paste it onto the picture of the slender person they want to become. Nothing is too far out if it helps you visualize and reach your goal!

4. Stay focused. Put "post it" notes with positive statements like, "I can do it!" "I will be 20 pounds lighter by___" on your bathroom mirror, car dashboard, on the refrigerator, etc.

5. Goal setting is a continual project. It is not just a one time resolution made on New Year's Day. Turn your resolutions into reality!

6. Symbols or objects that bring back the positive feelings of a past accomplishment, such as a photograph, trophy or award can boos confidence, self-esteem and motivation in the present moment. Keep reminder in eye's view and surround yourself with mementos of big events that represent personal success.

DARE TO SUCCEED!

THE OLD ADAGE, "If at first you don't succeed, try, try again" is familiar wisdom to the field of weight loss. As with all things in life, success generally follows a long line of "prior attempts" (which is the politically correct way of saying "past failures")! This brings to mind the record of a famous American. His message was, "Don't be afraid to fail."

- Failed in business—age 22
- Ran for legislature and was defeated—age 23
- Again failed in business—age 24
- Elected to legislature—age 25
- Sweetheart died—age 27
- Defeated for Speaker—age 29
- Defeated for Congress—age 34
- Defeated for Congress—age 37
- Defeated for Congress—age 39
- Defeated for Senate—age 46
- Defeated for Vice President—age 47
- Elected president of the United States—age 51

This man was Abraham Lincoln.

LOSE WEIGHT
WHILE YOU SLEEP

SCIENTISTS NOW SUGGEST that poor sleep habits may be as important as improper nutrition and physical inactivity in the development of chronic illness and obesity.

Up to 70 million Americans have some sort of a sleep disturbance that can be caused by emotional, environmental or physical factors, such as sleep apnea. The effect of sleep deprivation is profound. Right up there with food and water, sleep is a basic human need.

According to the National Sleep Foundation in Washington, D.C., one-third of the population sleeps 6.5 or fewer hours than the 8 hours sleep specialists recommend as optimal. Several recent studies demonstrated that sleeping 6.5 or fewer hours for successive nights caused potentially harmful metabolic, hormonal and immune changes.

Sleep researchers at the University of Chicago found that sleep deficits impaired the body's processing of the sugar, glucose, showing signs of insulin resistance in 50% of the volunteers. Other hormonal changes that promote weight gain were seen in the sleep-deprived, as well. Leptin, a hormone that signals satiety and regulates energy balance, can increase fat deposition, slow metabolism and over-stimulate the appetite if its level dips.

When held to 4 hours of sleep for a week, volunteers reported being hungrier than when they had adequate rest, and would overwhelmingly ask for candy, starchy foods and salty snacks, such as potato chips. There were no cravings for fruit and vegetables!

Whether millions of cases of obesity and diabetes could be prevented if U.S. citizens increased their sleep to 8 hours per night cannot yet be answered conclusively. There is evidence, though, that the extreme—6 hours or less per night—is not conducive for optimal health.

Consistently sleeping 7 to 8 hours per night not only aids one's health, mental acuity and attitude, it also improves one's appearance.

A study reported in *The Journal of Investigative Dermatology* found that inadequate sleep resulted in the skin being more vulnerable to allergens and bacteria with a slower recovery time for healing. Because sleep deprivation affects hormonal levels, skin can become dry, more prone to acne, and hair thinning or actual loss can result. Lack of sleep increases adrenaline, which can cause superficial blood vessels to constrict, creating an ashen complexion in darker skinned people or a pallid coloring of light skin. It appears Mom was correct when she said "you need your beauty sleep."

Of all the health prescriptions and weight-loss techniques available, wouldn't it be great if all it took to lose those extra pounds and get healthier was to turn off the alarm clock?

In Trying Times

WHEN IT SEEMS AS THOUGH THE WHOLE WORLD IS COMING APART at the seams, it is difficult to focus on health and nutrition. After the devastating events of September 11, 2001, for example, considering the hazards of transfats in the diet or tips on weight reduction just don't seem that important! Grief and fear hit us like a jet plane flying smack dab into our mid section…and it hurts.

We all need comfort during difficult times and food is a common thing to grab for its calming effect. Physiologically, carbohydrates spur our bodies to release the hormone serotonin, which makes us feel more relaxed. Fats can create a feeling of lethargy and sleepiness when eaten. Sales in the chocolate industry spiked dramatically after the World Trade Center Tragedy and have remained high. Long known as a major comfort food, chocolate melts at 98.6 degrees (our body temperature) creating a most pleasurable oral sensation.

When it seems as though you've lost all control with what goes into your mouth during stressful times, remember to be gentle with yourself and save the guilt trips! A few days of overeating have never made anyone fat. Weight problems occur quickly and easily when those "days" turn into weeks and months. Continued haphazard eating is when trouble sets in. Remember too, a steady diet of processed junk…candy, cookies, white flour/white sugar, etc…all wreak havoc on one's system and typically produce a depressive state. Simple carbohydrates, sugars, enter the bloodstream quickly elevating the insulin level then dropping the level just as rapidly, creating a crash which makes us feel exhausted. Abstain from sweets and processed foods for typically two weeks and the cravings will diminish greatly.

If you find yourself in a continual pattern of unconscious/uncontrolled eating please know there are many "less self-destructive" ways to relax the soul. Find support that will give you the guidance, motivation and reassurance needed to get back on a healthy track. When under stress, eating actually isn't the best way to deal with it. Physical movement, distraction by calling a friend or taking a hot bath work much better to relax the system.

As we enter these times of expanded awareness, let us commit ourselves even more deeply to making the world a kinder, safer place. It all begins within ourselves.

10 TIPS
TO CHANGE YOUR LIFE

1. Become committed to yourself; be your best friend.

2. Face your fears.

3. Take responsibility for your life.

4. Make your own sunlight and let yourself shine.

5. Do whatever it takes and do it now.

6. Learn to quiet your inner judge/critic by listening to your inner ally.

7. Think good thoughts.

8. Work harder on yourself than you do at your job.

9. Set "do-able" goals for an exercise plan, an "eating for health" regimen and a program for mental fitness.

10. Let love be your guiding force in all that you do and all that you are.

INSPIRATION

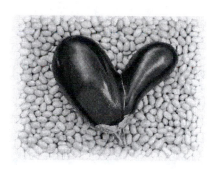

FEAR NOT

I T HAS BEEN SAID THAT THERE ARE TWO BASIC HUMAN EMOTIONS—
love and fear. Pleasure and pain are another way of saying the same thing. For
most of us, we want to stick with the love and pleasure side of life...nobody
wants to deal with pain and fear. Yet, in the human experience, it seems clear
we cannot have one without the other...love and fear go hand in hand.

Several years ago, my worst nightmare came true when my husband was diagnosed with terminal cancer. Previously so healthy and full of life, he died in my
arms after a six-month struggle with lymphoma...leaving me a 39-year-old
widow with a four-year-old child. There are no words to express the pain and
grief I felt.

Within a year of Jerry's passing, both his parents died, then my father died, as
did both my godparents, with whom I was very close. A few years later, Duchess
my dog and K.C. my cat, both whom I'd had for 20 years, passed away. Then, in
that very same year, my dear mother was diagnosed with metastatic breast cancer and died in the spring. I still miss her.

During this same time span, while driving down the winding mountain road
I live on, unbelievably I came upon a horrible accident where the driver was
trapped underneath the wreckage. I was holding his hand as he, too...passed away.

One after another, people I loved were leaving me. I lived with a lot of fear and
felt like "Chicken Little," with the sky caving in. When would all the dying stop?

Then one night I had a most profound dream. I was seated at a desk in a class-
room. My husband Jerry was standing near a large blackboard in the front of the
room. He wrote the letters **F-E-A-R** enormously on the board with chalk. Very
matter of factly, he pointed to the letters, one by one, saying they stood for **F**alse
Evidence **A**ppearing **R**eal. I laughed and said it could also mean **Fu*k**
Everything **A**nd **R**un!

Suddenly, I heard Bob Marley music playing in the background...the tune *Three Little Birds*, with the chorus, "Don't worry 'bout a thing, cuz ev'ry little thing's gonna be all right," repeating over and over. Jerry again pointed to each letter of F-E-A-R and looking me straight in the eyes, said..."**F**orgetting **E**verything's **A**ll **R**ight"... "**F**orgetting **E**verything's **A**ll **R**ight."

That dream was pivotal in my healing and freed me to the truth. To be able to fully love, we must accept the fact that with all life comes loss and impermanence. Paradoxically, once we embrace pain and fear as inevitable, life becomes less frightening and we are more capable of creating even deeper love and connection. Everything truly is "all right" when we rest in the arms of acceptance.

> *Come to the edge*
> *life said.*
> *They said:*
> *We are afraid.*
> *Come to the edge*
> *life said.*
> *They came.*
> *It pushed them...*
> *And they* **Flew.**
>
> ~Guillaume Apollinaire

POWERFUL CONVICTION

"**O**UR DEEPEST FEAR IS NOT THAT WE ARE INADEQUATE.
Our deepest fear is that we are powerful beyond measure.
It is our light, not our darkness, that most frightens us.
We ask ourselves, who am I to be brilliant, gorgeous, talented, fabulous?
Actually, who are you not to be? You are a child of God.
Your playing small does not serve the world.
There is nothing enlightened about shrinking
so that other people won't feel insecure around you.
We were born to make manifest the glory of God that is within us.
It is not just in some of us: it is in everyone.
And as we let our own light shine,
we unconsciously give other people permission to do the same.
As we are liberated from our own fear, our presence automatically liberates others."

Nelson Mandela, spoke some true words of wisdom in this 1994 inaugural speech. Life is too short not to let yourself shine. It all begins with our bodies and a positive attitude. What better time than **right now** to improve upon your health and exercise regimen?

LOVE

THE FOLLOWING SENTIMENT WAS READ AT MY WEDDING by the Reverend Ernlé Young of Stanford Memorial Church.

Love is a friendship that has caught fire.

It is quiet understanding, mutual confidence, sharing, and forgiving.

It is loyalty through good and bad.

It settles for less than perfection and makes allowances for human weaknesses.

Love is content with the present. It hopes for the future and does not brood over the past.

It's the day-in and day-out chronicles of irritations, problems, small disappointments, big victories, and working towards common goals.

If you have love in your life, it can make up for a great many things you lack.

If you don't have it—no matter what else there is…it is not enough.

So often we extend this level of compassion to others, but neglect to give it to ourselves. Those who suffer from food and weight issues often feel even less deserving. Commitment to a program of sound nutrition and exercise can be the first step towards showing one's self love and compassion, which is our birthright.

FEEDING THE SOUL

O
N A RECENT TRIP TO DISNEY WORLD IN ORLANDO, FLORIDA, I was struck by the number of severely overweight people I saw there. Again and again, I'd see folks so heavy they needed wheelchairs just to get around. I witnessed the plight of an obese woman who couldn't fit into her airplane seat. For seven hours she was strapped in a space far too small to accommodate her size. I hurt for her.

My purpose here is not to ridicule those challenged by excess weight—quite the contrary. My life's work has been to assist and support these people. I've used these examples as a backdrop for my real goal in discussing nutrition as a tool to enhance one's spirituality. Interest in matters of the soul are at an all time high. A recent cover story in Newsweek magazine reported that science and spirituality are having a revival of sorts and are coming together as never before.

In the bestselling book, *Talking to Heaven*, James Van Praagh states that the first step—the most basic element in becoming more open to one's soul—is to have a sound diet. The author went on to say the more pure the food, with very little or no refined sugars, caffeine or additives the better one's ability to connect with their inner being.

In the past, when I've made a steady diet of junk food, it has resulted in a disconnection from my own self—physically, mentally and emotionally. For me, being in an unconscious place doesn't serve to enlighten or expand my awareness. Having said all this, complete deprivation may not be spiritually healthy either. Another equally important side to "spiritual wellness" is *Balance*. Life is meant to bring joy and pleasure. It's okay to have a piece of birthday cake once in a while or even eat a whole bag of chips, if you feel that it will serve your emotional well being. Savor every bite without fear, guilt or judgement but think of these splurges as a "once in a while treat," rather than make a daily practice of it. Remember moderation is the key! Soulfood, whether healthy or not, can be a vital component to our spiritual development. It shows that we love and care for ourselves.

FOOD FOR THOUGHT

Aᴌᴌ ᴛʜᴏsᴇ ᴡᴇʟʟ-ɪɴᴛᴇɴᴅᴇᴅ, ʜᴇᴀʟᴛʜʏ ʀᴇsᴏʟᴜᴛɪᴏɴs made on January 1st often fizzle. Here are a few of my favorite quotes to keep up the motivation any time of the year.

- "Behold the turtle. He makes progress only when he sticks his neck out."

  James Conant

- "Whether you think you can or whether you think you can't—you're right."

  Henry Ford

- "Pain is inevitable. Suffering is optional." *Anonymous*

- "There are no short cuts to any place worth going." *Beverly Sills*

- "If you always do what you've always done then you'll always get what you've always gotten. If change is needed then you must do things differently." *Unknown*

- "There are no winners and losers, just winners and learners. Failure is an event, not a person." *The Healthy Way*

- "He who controls others is powerful, but he who masters himself is mightier still." *Lao Tzu*

- "Success comes in cans, failure comes in can'ts." *Mark Twain*

- "Life is what happens while you're busy making other plans." *John Lennon*

- "Never, never, never, never, never give up." *Winston Churchill*

- "Happiness is not the absence of problems—but rather the ability to deal with them." *Mark Twain*

- "You so often experience change, as though something terrible were happening, when in reality, the change is moving you from confinement in to freedom, from habit into truth. Crossroads are the call to exploration." *Emmanuel*

Dear Diary

October 14

Dear Diary,
I opened the kitchen cabinet
There is a candy bar
It speaks my name
Hand to mouth, without thought
I devour the sweetness
As soon as I swallow...Guilt sets in
I hate myself!
I am fat and ugly
It's a hopeless situation
Standing in front of the cabinet, I continue to eat

October 23

Dear Diary,
I opened the kitchen cabinet
There is a candy bar
It speaks my name
I pretend I don't see it
It yells out to me
Hand to mouth
I devour the sweetness
I can't believe I am in the same place
Before I swallow, Guilt sets in
I hate myself!
I am fat and ugly
It's such a hopeless situation
So I eat more

November 2

Dear Diary,

I opened the kitchen cabinet
There is a candy bar
It speaks my name
I grab it and eat it
It's a habit
I clearly see that I am addicted to sugar
I close the cabinet door
Before I eat more

November 10

Dear Diary,

I opened the kitchen cabinet
There is a candy bar
Before it speaks my name
I close the cabinet
I leave the kitchen and go for a walk

November 17

Dear Diary,

I don't buy candy bars anymore!

THE GIFT

A FEW YEARS AGO, I was involved in an experience that had a profound effect on my life. While driving down a winding mountain road, I came upon a horrendous accident. A 25-ton semi-truck had smashed into a thousand pieces and trapped underneath it all was the driver. From the wreckage he was able to grab my hand. Struggling for air, the driver begged, "Don't leave me." I assured him I would stay by his side. All my years as an ICU nurse made for an easy assessment. This man wasn't going to make it!

I asked his name. "Ron," he whispered.

I said, "Who do you love?"...

"Lori, my wife and Dana, my baby," he answered. With our hands tightly clutched, we prayed together. I told him I thought it was a good day to die and not to be scared.

I watched as he took his last breath. I felt him leave. As I held this strange dead man's hand, while knee deep in mud along the side of the road, I found myself experiencing a state of Bliss! I felt surrounded by light and a voice echoed in my head. I heard the words, "You are never alone. Even when you think you are, you are not and when you die, thousands of hands will reach for you. They reach out for everyone! There is a divine plan and reason for everything. Just Trust. Trust the process."

I will forever be grateful for my encounter with Ron, because in his dying, I have become more alive. The truth is, each one of us really only has just this moment in time, so we had better do it, say it, and be it today, because tomorrow is promised to no one.

So stop waiting until you lose 10 lbs., until you find the right mate, until you pay off all the bills, until winter is over—to realize the time is NOW. Set your fears aside, live like there's no tomorrow and be more compassionate to everyone you encounter, starting with yourself. Trust in the gift of the present moment.

LESSONS

I've learned that everyone's story is "To be Continued." We are all a work-in-progress.

I've learned sometimes you must give up the life you have planned, for the one that's waiting for you.

I've learned that we can have many lifetimes during our existence. Make at least one of them count.

I've learned if someone isn't buying you flowers—buy them for yourself.

I've learned that we are never, ever truly alone. Even when we think we are—we aren't. Trust it!

I've learned that no matter how thin you slice it—there are always two sides.

I've learned that there are no mistakes, just opportunities to learn from and love more.

I've learned that it takes a long time to become the person we want to be.

I've learned that you control your attitude or it controls you.

I've learned that our background and circumstances may have influenced who we are, but we are responsible for who we become.

I've learned that no matter the consequences, those who are honest with themselves get further in life.

I've learned that the sky is not the limit!

STRUGGLE

A DVERSITY, AND THE STRUGGLE THAT RESULTS, is intimately connected to life and can often be a doorway to transformation. In my years of caring for cancer patients who endured unimaginable pain and loss; and from witnessing **Healthy Way** clients who live with enormous shame and guilt; it appears suffering is a universal law and necessary for growth.

A while back my daughter received a "butterfly kit" for her birthday, and from it we both learned an incredible lesson in the value of struggle. We put the cardboard butterfly house together, complete with plastic windows for viewing, and sent away for the worms which were guaranteed to change into cocoons and then emerge as live butterflies within a few weeks. It was fascinating to watch the whole process, and sure enough, we released a dozen beautiful new born butterflies and felt giddy as we watched our babies fly away. But one of them didn't make it. Not knowing any better, when the first butterfly showed signs of emerging and was struggling to get out...my daughter took a pair of manicuring scissors and snipped the cocoon open. The butterfly emerged easily but looked deformed and was never able to spread its wings. Instead of developing as the other butterflies did into a creature free to fly, the poor soul we tampered with, spent its brief life looking like an elongated pill bug.

The struggle necessary to pass through the tiny opening of the cocoon actually forces fluid from the body into the wings...an essential part of the process.

I think Elizabeth Kubler-Ross, M.D., said it best:

"If we could see that everything—
sadness, pain, struggle, even tragedy
were gifts in disguise,
we would then find
the best way to nourish the soul."

TIME IN A BOTTLE

I T IS AMAZING TO REALLY COME TO TERMS, or at least realize, the fact that "none of us will make it off the planet alive!" Death is often viewed as an inconvenience or problem to be dealt with by our age-defying society. In America, dying is something that is hidden away. Even our language about it reflects avoidance…we "expire;" the patient "terminated;" "he was lost on the table."

During my bedside nursing days, I found the dying patients to actually be the most *alive*. They said what they thought and didn't waste time because they knew their days were numbered. If all of us were wise enough to live in that state of being, perhaps just 50% of the time, our lives would be filled with much more joy and less regret.

Here is a thought-provoking exercise, aimed at living life more consciously:

The average life expectancy in the U.S. is about 75 years. If you multiply 75 years by 52 weeks in a year, the answer is 3,900…which is the number of weekends that the average person has in their entire lifetime.

Whatever age you are right now, subtract that from 75, then multiply that by 52 and the answer will reflect how many weekends you have left in life to enjoy.

At 45 years old, I have 1,560 weekends to go if I have a typical life expectancy.

As a visual symbol of the weekends remaining in your life, get a large-size clear container and inside it put pennies, pebbles, marbles, beans—whatever small token you'd like, in the amount of weekends you have left. Then, as each weekend approaches, take one out and throw it away.

What a dramatic way to gain greater insight into the fleeting nature of life, by watching our time here on earth diminish! The goal is to help us all live better, and in the process, to help us die better, as well.

ANNA JEAN

ANNA JEAN WAS A CONSCIENTIOUS **HEALTHY WAY** CLIENT, who was one of those great teachers of life's many lessons. Negative self-talk is common amongst most people, however, for Anna Jean it was severe. She hated her body, her complexion was never clear enough, and she called every day a "bad hair day."

Actually she was an attractive woman with a heart of gold, but her generosity extended to others, rather than to herself. Anna Jean suffered from not feeling "good enough" about her self-worth. She had a distorted perspective and obsession with her appearance.

My fellow counselors and I expended lots of energy trying to get Anna Jean to see the truth and relax her insecurities, but eventually she stopped coming in.

Several years later, Anna Jean came back in to **The Healthy Way.** Things in her life were much different, as she had suffered a debilitating stroke. The left side of her body was partially paralyzed, causing her eye and mouth to droop. Her left arm had limited movement, and she walked with the aid of a cane.

Amazingly, the stroke forced Anna Jean to have a magnificent awakening—a true epiphany! She said her idea of what was important in life had been forever altered. She was truly transformed and no longer obsessed with her appearance.

"I drool now," she joked. "I am happy just to get out of bed every day. I don't have the time, energy or desire to berate myself anymore. I am grateful to have my family and *my life*."

As she spoke, the beauty and radiance that shone from her very being almost took my breath away.

I believe each of us is born into this world with a deep sense of unconditional love for ourselves. For many, this love diminishes when our innate creativity and sense of wonder collide with the conformity of daily living. What ensues is a disconnection to self and the seeds of fear and insecurity take root.

So often, in the process of being human, only after we have suffered some enormous loss do we return to a place of compassion for ourselves and others. Anna Jean was a perfect example of this.

She sent me a thank-you card some time after our visit, saying her physical condition was steadily improving. She didn't need to mention her mental attitude, because the quote on the front of her card said it all...

> *Be content with what you have,*
> *Rejoice in the way things are.*
> *When you realize there is nothing lacking,*
> *the whole world belongs to you.*
>
> ~Lao Tzu

INDEX